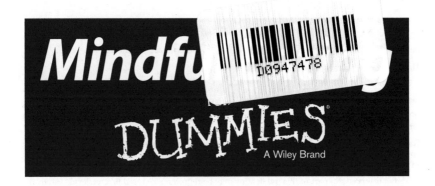

Mindfulness

DUMMIES
A Wiley Brand

by Laura Dawn, RHN

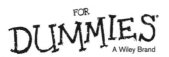

FOR
DUMMIES
A Wiley Brand

Mindful Eating For Dummies®

Published by: **John Wiley & Sons, Ltd.,** The Atrium, Southern Gate, Chichester, www.wiley.com

This edition first published 2014

© 2014 John Wiley & Sons, Ltd, Chichester, West Sussex.

Registered office

John Wiley & Sons Ltd, The Atrium, Southern Gate, Chichester, West Sussex, PO19 8SQ, United Kingdom

For details of our global editorial offices, for customer services and for information about how to apply for permission to reuse the copyright material in this book please see our website at www.wiley.com.

Wiley publishes in a variety of print and electronic formats and by print-on-demand. Some material included with standard print versions of this book may not be included in e-books or in print-on-demand. If this book refers to media such as a CD or DVD that is not included in the version you purchased, you may download this material at http://booksupport.wiley.com. For more information about Wiley products, visit www.wiley.com.

Designations used by companies to distinguish their products are often claimed as trademarks. All brand names and product names used in this book are trade names, service marks, trademarks or registered trademarks of their respective owners. The publisher is not associated with any product or vendor mentioned in this book.

For general information on our other products and services, please contact our Customer Care Department within the U.S. at 877-762-2974, outside the U.S. at (001) 317-572-3993, or fax 317-572-4002. For technical support, please visit www.wiley.com/techsupport.

For technical support, please visit www.wiley.com/techsupport.

A catalogue record for this book is available from the British Library.

ISBN 978-1-118-87768-5 (pbk); ISBN 978-1-118-87769-2 (ebk); ISBN 978-1-118-87770-8 (ebk)

Printed in Great Britain by TJ International, Padstow, Cornwall.

10 9 8 7 6 5 4 3 2 1

Contents at a Glance

Table of Contents

Introduction

I'll never forget the moment, many years ago, that I reached down to the ground, snapped a nicely sized asparagus stalk at its base and bit the tip off. I was wrestling with the preconceived notion that I didn't even like asparagus. That notion was completely shattered as a burst of juice flooded my mouth unlike anything that I ever expected. This was *real* food, *fresh* food – and the first major blessing and break-through in my life, as I was mostly raised on packaged foods, like so many of us were (and still are). And the second break-through was that I was present to experience it. In a sense, it was the total awe of this unexpected sensory experience that launched me into the present moment, and with that came my total love affair with real food *and* with the practice of discovering how to eat it more mindfully.

Even after I shifted my dietary habits and fell in love with whole, real, fresh foods and went from reaching for chips to reaching for a smoothie – a major step in the right direction – I kept notic-ing that although I was reaching for healthier foods, I still had a strong tendency to reach for them in an automatic way, without fully tuning in to the inner awareness of my body. Even though I was full, I still felt unsatisfied and wanted more – one of the many examples of the way mindlessness affected my life.

When I started implementing mindfulness practices and more specifically mindful eating, a radical shift occurred in my life. I saw that my relationship with food was the reflection of my relationship with life, and this inspired a huge shift in the way I experienced food, my body and my life in general. The act of eating a single cherry would make me so excited, so struck by awe and wonder, that I wanted to shout my excitement from the rooftops! I knew that as I embarked on the path to becom-ing a holistic nutritionist these mindfulness practices would be invaluable tools not only for myself, but also for my clients as well – and they've now proven themselves a million times over.

This book is the result of years of practice, study and teaching, and was the next step in introducing mindful eating to a wider audience and anyone interested in exploring their own relationship with food.

About this Book

The practice of mindful eating and all that it entails is a journey that provides you with an opportunity to discover a very special relationship with food; one that you have the pleasure and privilege to experience and claim as your own.

Mindful Eating For Dummies offers you many tips, tools, suggestions and exercises rooted in the practice of mindfulness to help you uncover and explore your relationship with food. This mindful exploration can be a catalyst for profound change; it can transform a challenging relationship with food into an enjoyable one that supports your health and fosters your happiness.

This book is laid out as a reference guide, with each chapter standing alone, so after you peruse the Table of Contents feel free to jump to the chapter that calls to you the most. The sidebars offer complementary and supporting content that you can skip over or delve into for extra information.

Foolish Assumptions

Every day that I sat down to write this book, I thought of you, yes, *you*, and who you are, what you're like and what your primary concerns are. In order to reach you with the information that would benefit you the most, I had to make a few assumptions about you:

- ✔ You feel like you struggle with your relationship with food and want to find a healthy balance, but you don't know where to start.
- ✔ You've heard about some of the benefits of mindful eating, but you're not exactly sure what it actually is.

✔ You're interested in how mindful eating can help you lose weight, manage a chronic disease, end chronic overeating, find greater enjoyment from food or work with a disordered relationship with food and eating.

✔ You're interested in fostering a healthier relationship with your body.

✔ You're willing to try the practices in this book before you decide whether they can benefit you or not.

✔ You're not afraid to try something new, and you're open to what new experiences may teach you.

✔ You want to discover how to approach eating from a lifestyle rather than a diet approach.

✔ You're a healthcare or holistic practitioner who would like to introduce mindful eating to your patients and clients.

Icons Used in This Book

Icons are weaved into this book as the *For Dummies* way of drawing your attention to and highlighting important information.

This icon is worthy of your attention. It informs you of special advice to help you recall key principles from the chapter.

When you come across this icon, be open and ready to try something new. You may be guided through a mindful eating technique or engage with an exercise in your mindful eating journal (discussed in Chapter 4) to help you better understand the practice and principles of mindfulness and mindful eating.

Pay special attention to the note next to this icon. It cautions you against potential problems and helps you avoid them.

Soak in the meaningful words from the wise offered next to this icon.

Beyond the Book

In addition to the wealth of material offered in the book that you're reading right now, you can also access additional resources online. Check out extra articles about mindful eating at www.dummies.com/extras/mindfuleating.

Changing habitual patterns around food and eating can take some time. One of the best ways to help you form new habits is by asking yourself questions like: 'Am I hungry?' Visit www.dummies.com/cheatsheet/mindfuleating to find the Cheat Sheet to help you navigate this and other questions with grace and ease and to strengthen your mindful eating muscles.

Where to Go from Here

This book is laid out in a modular way so that you can dive in wherever you want to start exploring. Perhaps you'd like to have a good look at the Table of Contents and use your intuition to start wherever you feel called.

If you're new to mindful eating, I recommend you take a more traditional approach and start with Part I. Chapter 1 lays a solid foundation for you to build on, and then you can read the chapters in order after that, or in whatever way you feel is appropriate for you. Each chapter complements the others, yet offers standalone material and information to aid you on your mindful eating journey.

Part I

Getting Started with Mindful Eating

In this part . . .

✔ You are introduced to mindful eating and its roots in the practice of mindfulness.

✔ You find out about the many ways that people eat mindlessly and how mindfulness can help prevent some of the negative consequences of eating without paying attention.

✔ You identify how mindful eating can help you as you discover the wonderful benefits that mindfulness and mindful eating have to offer.

Chapter 1

Discovering Mindful Eating

*A*t first glance, mindful eating may sound simple. And at its most basic level, it *is* simple, yet mindful eating is also extremely profound and goes far beyond merely slowing down or removing distractions while you eat.

In this chapter I lay the groundwork for the chapters to come by exploring in-depth what mindful eating actually is, uncovering its roots in the art and practice of mindfulness, and looking at who can benefit the most from incorporating mindful eating into their everyday lives.

Exploring the Different Slices of the Mindful Eating Pie

To help you understand what mindful eating is and how it can help you, check out the opposite side of the coin and examine a few *mindless eating* scenarios. See if you can identify with any or all of the following situations:

  ✓ Can you remember a time when you walked up to your fridge, opened the door, picked out some leftovers and started eating them without really paying attention to what you were doing, as if you were on some kind of automatic pilot? And then all of a sudden you clued back in, realized what you were doing and noticed that half the food was already gone, but you only vaguely remembered tasting it.

✔ What about this scenario: you walk into your kitchen and there it is, in plain sight on the counter – the chocolate cake. You ate two pieces of that chocolate cake yesterday, felt subpar afterwards and told yourself that you wouldn't do that again. But today's a new day . . . and that's a new piece of cake! You go back and forth in your mind, struggling with the lure of the cake, and before you know it, you're eating another piece of cake faster than you'd like to admit while feelings of guilt, shame and blame start to arise before the last bite is gone.

✔ Can you remember a time you continued to eat so much food your stomach hurt, even though you knew you would regret it shortly afterwards?

✔ Do you ever notice other things often distract you while you eat? Perhaps you routinely eat (and often overeat) without paying attention to what you're doing because you're distracted by a movie, a conversation over dinner or preoccupied with emails while working at your desk. Afterwards you're left feeling unsatisfied and wanting more, despite being full.

✔ Have you ever eaten something and noticed that before you were even finished eating it, you were already lost in thoughts of how you wanted more of that food and had started mentally planning how you were going to get it?

✔ Do you ever turn to food as a means of avoiding an uncomfortable situation or because you're procrastinating on a project, or simply because you feel bored? What about after an argument with a friend or your partner? Ever notice yourself automatically turning to the pleasure of food as a means of distracting yourself from feeling something you'd rather not feel?

✔ What about using food as a pick-me-up from the pressures of leading a busy and stressful life, or as a way to wake yourself up when you're feeling tired or run down?

Whatever is the case for you, the common thread here is a tendency towards mindless eating, the antidote to which is mindful eating – the topic of this book.

At mindless times like these you can benefit from the practice of mindfulness, which helps you to snap out of that all-too-familiar knee-jerk reaction mode (see cake, eat cake) into conscious-choice mode (does my body really want cake right now? How will I feel after I eat this?).

This book is a guide to help you step out of the mindless eating patterns that most everyone is familiar with and into a way of living that cultivates mindfulness as its foundation and incorporates mindful eating as a solution to many of the food-related troubles so many people experience.

Who Can Benefit from Mindful Eating?

The wonderful part about mindful eating is that it can benefit anyone and everyone. No matter how old you are, what you do, where you live, how active you are or how much you weigh, everyone can reap the rewards of eating more mindfully.

Mindful eating can be especially helpful to you if:

- ✔ You notice you regularly eat when you're not hungry.
- ✔ You've tried many different diets with little success.
- ✔ You struggle with being over- or underweight.
- ✔ Your health is having a negative impact on other areas of your life, including your relationships.
- ✔ Your health is causing you pain, suffering or general discontent.
- ✔ Your health is preventing you from living the life you truly want to be living.
- ✔ You're constantly thinking about food and what you should or shouldn't be eating.
- ✔ You feel uncomfortable in your body.

✔ You want to discover how to become more mindful about your food choices.

✔ You regularly eat to cover up your emotions.

✔ You eat as a method of distraction.

✔ You're afraid to eat from fear of gaining weight.

✔ You're afraid to eat in front of other people.

✔ You want to feel better about and more accepting of your body.

✔ You feel that you're too busy to eat healthfully.

Indulging in the richness of mindful eating

At the most basic level, mindful eating is simply *paying attention* while you eat. It may sound simple, yet this seemingly mundane task has the capacity to offer you a vast array of life-changing insights and has enough depth to keep you busy exploring new territory for at least a lifetime!

At this point, you may be asking yourself: what am I supposed to be paying attention to? Great question! To which there are innumerable answers! When it comes to where you choose to place your awareness, you have a buffet of choices that can be divided into two fundamental categories:

✔ Your inner reality

✔ Your outer reality

Exploring the world around you

One of the joys of living is being able to experience the world around you through your senses; by touching, seeing, smelling, tasting and hearing life, you have the opportunity to explore countless experiences through your senses. Using the full range of your senses is one of the easiest techniques at your immediate disposal to practice mindfulness.

Put down this book for a moment and close your eyes. What do you hear? The art and act of listening is enough to ground you in this moment. See how long you can listen before your mind steps in to label the experience. Try to have a direct experience with the sounds without the need to identify what they are (bird, cars, dog barking and so on). When thoughts do arise, just notice the thoughts without adding another layer of labeling on top of that, as if you're watching your thoughts pass by like clouds in the sky and continuously bring your attention back to the direct experience of listening.

This was your first mindfulness practice. How did it feel? What did you notice? I'll dive into mindfulness a little further along in the chapter, so stay *tuned in* – literally!

When it comes to eating, you can have a whole new experience of food through the simple practices of becoming mindful of your sensory experience before, during and after you eat. This practice of mindfulness includes paying attention to the taste, smell, sight, sound and touch, as well as the *mouthfeel* (the way food feels in your mouth), of food. You can choose to focus on many aspects of your senses, but one of the most important things to remember is that the gifts of these unique experiences are all fleeting and require awareness and attention towards them. Otherwise these gifts pass by without you registering that they even happened. You don't get to experience them, and that means you're missing out on life. All of these sensory experiences are occurring in the present moment, which makes tuning into your senses a technique that anchors you to the gift of here and now.

Chapter 9 provides a more in-depth look at experiencing food through your senses.

Welcoming the universe within

Think of your senses as the doorway that connects your outer reality to your inner reality. Your *interpretation* of the world that you experience around you with all of your senses makes your experience unique to you. The way you perceive, process and filter your reality through your thoughts, feelings and emotions makes up your personal experience of life. Twenty people can attend the same dinner event and all have a completely different experience based on the way that they experienced the food, their social interactions and even the surrounding environment.

In addition to paying attention to your outer reality with your senses, mindful eating invites you to explore your thoughts, feelings, cravings and emotions surrounding food and eating. When it comes to eating something, you may think to yourself, 'I've tasted that a million times before! I know what that tastes like,' and without realizing it, you've defined your experience before you've even had it! When practicing mindful eating, you allow yourself to approach food and eating as though every experience is a new experience. This kind of attitude helps you stay open to new information that may guide you in a new direction, a direction of your own choosing.

A vast universe within awaits you. That's the beauty of mindfulness. It opens the doorway to the exploration of one of the greatest journeys of all – discovering your own self.

Take a moment to close your eyes and imagine a slice of pizza. What are the first thoughts that come to mind? Your initial thoughts may be: fattening, delicious, guilt, tempting, addiction, control, out-of-control, pleasure and so on.

The practice of mindful eating allows you to notice your thoughts around food and become more aware of all the judgments and belief systems that you bring to the table when you eat. Pizza is just pizza, but *you* define how you experience it. Better yet, through mindful awareness, you can start to notice your thoughts about food with an attitude of non-judgment and notice how your thoughts are shaping your experience. Chapter 5 has more on cultivating a mindful eating mindset.

I had a client who would think about food, particularly ice cream and cookies, for most of her day. She expressed how it made her feel bad about herself and also how much it got in the way of her work. Ironically, when she would go home and eat cookies and ice cream she was so preoccupied with thoughts of guilt and worry that she was rarely present to actually experience eating what she thought about eating all day long!

Mindful eating can be viewed as a way to train your mind to become present so that you can have a more joyful experience with eating and with life in general. The present moment has so much to offer you, especially when it comes to enjoying the simply delicious pleasures of food. You'll enjoy your food more thoroughly after you begin to stay present long enough to really experience it!

Lastly, when it comes to exploring the universe within you, mindful eating also helps you tune into your actual physical inner reality, including chewing, swallowing, digesting, how food makes you feel physically after you eat and how your body feels before you eat. The body scan practice outlined in Chapter 8 is a great way to help you start tuning into this wonderful world within and start benefiting from getting to know yourself a little bit better.

Serving up a broader definition of mindful eating

Although the term mindful eating refers to the act of eating and paying attention while you eat to both your inner and outer reality, the larger concept extends out beyond this. Mindful eating includes the moments leading up to eating as well as the moments after eating (and everything in between!) that envelop the whole process of eating.

Your relationship with food reflects and encompasses your relationship to yourself, including the exploration of your thinking mind, your feeling body and the energy underlying your emotions. On the highest level, getting to know and understand your relationship with food can be a reflection of your relationship with life itself.

Take a sneak peak at some of the wonderful things that you can discover by cultivating mindful eating, and which are explored throughout this book. Mindful eating:

✔ Tunes you into your hunger and fullness cues so that you can use your inner wisdom to choose the appropriate amount of food for you that is satisfying, nourishing and supports your health and optimal weight.

✔ Reconnects you to the inherent wisdom that you already possess.

✔ Empowers you with the freedom to consciously choose what you eat.

✔ Helps you become aware of what's triggering you to eat when you are and when you aren't hungry.

✔ Helps you become more aware of how your food choices are affecting your physical, mental and spiritual wellbeing.

✔ Encourages you to become aware of how your food choices affect the environment.

✔ Allows you to be present with the food you're eating in order to appreciate the moment-to-moment experience and enjoyment of food.

✔ Teaches you how to engage all of your senses while eating to fully experience the act of eating.

✔ Offers insights into your relationship with food, your body and with life.

✔ Shines the light of awareness on your food-related thoughts, judgments and belief systems.

✔ Involves a wide range of tools, techniques and practices to help you cultivate awareness of your relationship with food.

✔ Cultivates a specific, positive mindset that can have a far reaching impact on all areas of your life.

✔ Helps you become aware of mindless eating tendencies and develop new ways of relating to food that avoid the (often painful) consequences of eating without paying attention.

Think of mindful eating as less a specific practice and more as a set of tools that you can use on your mindful eating journey. Mindful eating then becomes part of a broader mindful lifestyle where you're cultivating awareness in the everyday moments of your life.

Looking at the pleasure – and pain – of eating

Food, and the act of eating it, offers an incredible source of pleasure in life. Yet, for a surprising number of people, food – or rather, their underlying relationship with food – is a major cause of struggle, pain and suffering. Why is this?

Paradoxically, western culture is one of the most health-obsessed cultures in the world, yet at the same time it is extremely unhealthy, with an unprecedented increase in rates of food-related diseases and obesity, especially amongst the young.

In today's culture, navigating the media hype related to food is difficult. On the one hand the media is constantly presenting images of slim and skinny celebrities, new dieting gimmicks and products that offer a more beautiful future. And on the other hand, everywhere you look you see unhealthy, packaged, processed and addictive foods dangling in front of you, whether you're watching TV, surfing the internet, standing at the checkout counter of your local grocery store or being bombarded with billboard images of unhealthy foods. Never before in the history of the world has there been more than a billion people starving and simultaneously more than a billion people overweight – what extremes!

On top of that, more people than ever before are unhappy with the shape and size of their bodies and are continuously striving to meet a culturally defined definition of beauty. In a weight-obsessed culture where food plays a large role in how much you weigh, it's no wonder that so many people struggle with their relationship with food.

Many people aim their frustration and discontent towards food – but food is just an innocent bystander! Food doesn't cause you suffering; food is simply food. In itself, food is neither good nor bad. Rather, the way people *relate* to food causes much of their distress. When you *mindlessly* relate to your food, your thoughts, judgments, opinions, belief systems and busy mind cloud and obscure your experience. And unfortunately, what could be a satisfying, enjoyable relationship turns into a never-ending uphill battle.

Taking a Holistic Approach

In the past, people's obsession with health tended to be quite food-centric, with a focus on dieting, thinness and weight loss, and with the never-ending quest for the holy grail of youth and beauty. Recently there has been a gradual shift toward a bigger, more all-encompassing definition of health. This larger framework incorporates a more integrated mind-body-spirit approach to health and looks at all aspects of health and wellness. This holistic approach has placed an increased focus on the many health-related benefits of mindfulness and meditation, which originated from the eastern wisdom traditions such as Buddhism but are now commonplace in western culture.

With this holistic framework in mind, a more integrated approach to food choices can be applied. You will discover that not only *what* you eat, but also *how* you eat and *why* you eat influences your health.

Although mindful eating is more focused on *how* and *why* you eat rather than on *what* you eat, you may also notice a gradual shift in *what* you eat as a by-product of becoming more aware of *how* and *why* you eat. Make sense? You can then utilize mindful eating as a method of discovering which foods feel best to you and your body.

Discovering a healthy relationship with food

At the core of mindful eating is an exploration of your relationship with food, allowing you to gain awareness and insight into how this relationship is affecting you, your health and, ultimately, your life. The practice of mindful eating allows you to see food as something that you're connected to, sustained by and in relationship with, something that supports the totality of your health, including your mind, body and spirit.

Now for the big question: is this relationship one that is supportive of your health and well-being? Or is it hindering your ability to blossom and flourish as the beautiful being that you are and preventing you from living the life you really want to live?

Essentially, one of the core intentions of exploring mindful eating is so that you can develop a *healthy relationship* with food. A relationship that is:

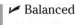

- Balanced
- Grateful

- ✔ Harmonious
- ✔ Inspiring
- ✔ Joyful
- ✔ Nourishing
- ✔ Pleasurable
- ✔ Satisfying
- ✔ Supportive

Does this sound like the kind of relationship you'd like to have with food? Is this noticeably different than the relationship you currently have? Through starting to eat mindfully, you can become aware of the places within your relationship with food that are out of alignment. You can then take the necessary steps to restore the balance and joy to your relationship with food that is not only incredibly rewarding, but is also your birthright to experience.

Think about yourself, your food and your eating habits in terms of a relationship. In the same way that your relationships with people can be highly complex, so too can be your relationship with food. What is your relationship with eating? On a piece of paper or in your mindful eating journal (flip to Chapter 4 for more on starting a mindful eating journal) contemplate your relationship with food and eating by asking yourself the following questions: does this relationship bring you pleasure? Does it cause you pain? Is it an abusive relationship? Is it a source of hardship and struggle or do you find it very easy to navigate what, how much and when to eat? Does this relationship cause you anxiety and stress? In general, does this relationship leave you feeling satisfied and nourished or usually wanting or desiring more? Is this a trusting relationship? Do you have confidence in this relationship? If you had to describe your relationship with food in one word, what would that word be?

Reflecting a larger relationship

Mindful eating encompasses the underlying relationship that you have with your food. When you delve deeper into this relationship you discover that it's made up of various and interconnected components. Primarily, your relationship with food includes your relationship with:

- **Eating:** the process by which you consume food.

- **Your body:** Much of the time, your eating habits stem directly from how you feel about your body. Your body shares a very intimate relationship with food: it's an aspect of nature that you willingly ingest into your body, merging your outer environment with your inner environment, literally becoming one with your food source – intimate indeed!

- **Your sense of self (incorporating aspects of the mental, emotional and spiritual):** many of your eating habits stem from how you feel about yourself, how worthy you feel you are and how much love and attention you give yourself.

- **Life itself:** Food sustains you in your life. Without food you wouldn't be able to experience the full range of life experiences that are such incredible gifts. The way you relate to food is a microcosm of how you relate to life.

Much of the mindful eating discussion that follows in the remainder of this book can help illuminate the aspects of your relationship to your body that may also need mindful attention, care and love. This process is about finding harmonious alignment within your relationship to your body, yourself, your food source and the earth.

Building a Solid Foundation: Delving into Mindfulness

By now, I'm sure you've noticed that the common thread weaving together the various aspects of mindful eating mentioned thus far is mindfulness, a large topic in itself and worthy of its own introduction. *Mindfulness* is the simple act of paying attention to whatever is arising in the present moment. Mindfulness is a heightened state of involvement and engagement with the present moment. The practice of mindfulness allows you to be actively alert and in a wakeful state and welcomes in an openness to new and continuously unfolding experiences.

Mindfulness is the underlying foundation in many different kinds of meditation practices, including sitting meditation, walking meditation and eating meditation too. Everything in life can be viewed and approached with the intention of mindfulness. Meditation isn't only reserved for yogis sitting in the lotus position. You can start to view every time you eat as a meditation in its own right, essentially the essence of what mindful eating is.

Mindfulness includes two primary components; the *what* and the *how*:

- ✓ **What you're doing:** You're paying attention and bringing awareness to your immediate experience.

- ✓ **How you're doing it:** You're paying attention with an attitude of openness, curiosity, compassion, acceptance and non-judgment towards your experience. Think of this as the mindset you're paying attention with. (Chapter 5 explores this mindset further.)

When you're being mindful, you observe the world around you with an immense amount of curiosity and openness to whatever is unfolding in the here and now. The key part about mindfulness is that on top of staying open, aware and curious you're also not judging, only noticing. By letting go of judgment, you can have a direct experience of reality without the moment being skewed and distorted by your thoughts.

You may be thinking: 'But I'm not a judgmental person!' Try to think of judgment more in terms of labeling everything you see. Judging goes hand in hand with thinking as humans are naturally wired to constantly evaluate their surroundings. (Check out Chapter 5 for more on judging.)

Dropping the speech balloon

I once heard well-known meditation teacher and renowned author Pema Chödrön describe mindfulness as 'dropping the speech balloon'. What she means by this is that you bear witness to what's occurring without having to label and attach thoughts to what's happening. You tend to constantly judge and label things: 'good' or 'bad', 'right' or 'wrong', 'appropriate' or 'inappropriate', 'I want it', 'I don't want it', 'I like it', 'I don't like it', and on and on it goes.

Strawberry savior

There once was a student who felt worried and anxious about life and sought guidance from an elderly monk. The monk listened to the student express worry about his future and responded with a short story that went like this:

'One day a Buddhist monk was walking through the mountains when all of a sudden a tiger jumped out at him and chased him towards the edge of a cliff. Hanging on to a vine, the monk skirted down to a ledge on the cliff only to see more tigers circulating below him in anticipation of his fall – and their dinner. As he searched for options, with tigers both above and below him, the monk looked over and glistening in the sun saw a magnificent, plump, bright red strawberry.

In that moment he is totally present, struck by awe for the beauty of the strawberry and mindfully reaches over and eats it carefully. "Wow!" he exclaimed. "What a delicious strawberry!"'

This story is a testament to how you can live your life amongst all the chaos – tigers above and tigers below – with mindful awareness. In some ways, you're in this predicament all the time, never fully knowing when your own life will come to an end. So what you can do is enjoy the moments that come to you, the moments that bring a sense of contentment, like eating a strawberry or watching a sunrise that you're fully present for.

Mindfulness allows you to witness the world around you with awe and wonder, like seeing the world around you through the eyes of a child without the incessant need to think, categorize and label everything that's happening. This grounded and present way of living prevents you from constantly being swept away on the thought train to a non-existent time in the past or the future.

Through mindfulness you discover how to become less reactive and how to respond to life with more thoughtfulness, a very helpful tool to have at your disposal when approaching your relationship with food amongst the chaos of everyday life. (Check out the sidebar 'Strawberry savior' for more on how to live with mindfulness, whatever the situation!)

Observing the observer

Mindfulness allows you to step back, so-to-speak, and become a conscious observer of your own life. This profound practice can help you make important distinctions when thoughts, emotions and sensations are occurring and help you differentiate between identifying them compared to identifying *with* them. This is the difference between noticing and observing a sad emotion rather than identifying with the emotion and feeling it as part of you. Instead of 'I am sad', approach it as, 'I am noticing a sad feeling at the moment'; notice a food craving rather than identify it as what you are in that moment. By staying open and curious about the ever-changing experiences of life, you can shift your attitude to approach something like a craving by thinking, 'Oh, isn't that interesting? Look how I'm reacting to this food in this moment,' rather than spiraling into thoughts of wanting or craving and identifying with this experience.

Think of it as if you're watching an actor on the stage – and that actor is you! Rather than identifying yourself as the actor, you step out of your role and watch yourself from a distance – essentially, observing the observer!

Training the puppy

As I already mentioned, the practice of mindfulness has a lot to do with training the mind. When you start to observe your mind, you may not be thrilled about what you see. That's okay. The mind often acts like a little puppy, constantly jumping all over the place, and it can be hard to control. You need to take a compassionate approach on this journey towards mindfulness.

Mindfulness is not about controlling your mind. The more you try to control your mind, the more it will resist conforming to the idea or notion of how you think it should be behaving. Mindfulness allows whatever thoughts arise to exist without judging or controlling anything. View your thoughts as clouds in the sky. Instead of trying to dictate the shape or direction of the clouds, you just watch them come and go with curiosity, openness and mindful awareness.

Think of training your mind like training a cute little puppy. Puppies rarely listen or sit still; they shred up the toilet paper or chew up your socks or pee all over the carpet, yet it's hard not to love them! If you get angry at the puppy for simply being a puppy and you're too hard on it, the puppy may grow up to rebel and misbehave, and grow into a mean dog that bites other people. The other approach is to train the puppy with loving-kindness, compassion, friendliness, care, mindful attention, playfulness, openness and focused attention. This method of training the puppy is more likely to be conducive to raising a mature dog that knows how to sit, stay, listen and behave in a friendly way.

Focusing on the gift of the present moment

Quite literally, now is the only moment that you have; it's the only time that you have to live in. All you have are these 'now' moments, for you to notice, experience, be with, and then let go of and welcome in the never-ending, continuous cycle of 'next' moments. Each moment is completely fresh and new and has never happened before and will never happen again. Isn't that amazing? What an incredible gift!

Moments arise, over and over again, that offer you a completely special and unique opportunity to experience them. Something happens in a moment and that same moment, no matter how much you want it to (or don't want it to), will never happen again.

This experience is reflected in the saying: *This too shall pass.*

Every single moment is a new moment, and despite your natural and human tendency to resist change, this is actually really good news. Only through the present moment do you have the opportunity to experience the greatest pleasures of your life – the smell of a flower, the taste of a fresh, juicy fruit, holding a sleeping baby in your arms. But if you're always focusing on the past or future then you miss out on the very precious moments that make up your life.

However, instead of relishing the gift of each moment, this simple truth is so easy to forget! It's as if you're sitting on the most precious gift in the world, yet you don't even realize that it's there! You get caught up in the struggle of life and all the while, right under your nose, is the most wonderful opportunity to experience the most valuable gift that you have access to.

Most of our suffering is rooted in two simple truths in relation to the present moment, both involving mindlessness. Instead of honoring, respecting, enjoying and experiencing this gift, you tend to:

✔ **Avoid, distract or move away from the present moment:** This distancing from the present moment may include a rejection or resistance to whatever is arising in the now as well as simply being lost in thought or distracted. You may dwell in the past or worry about the future.

✔ **Cling to the present moment:** This clinging involves resisting the change of the present moment into the next moment and not wanting to let it go by controlling, grasping or clinging to it. Again, your thoughts may be rooted in the past or future.

Try this simple mindfulness practice: sit down, cross-legged on the floor or comfortably in a chair, and focus your awareness on your breath. Every time you notice a thought pop into your mind, notice what the nature of that particular thought is. Tap your left knee if the thought is based in the past and tap your right knee if the thought is based in the future. Engage in this practice for five minutes. After you're done, notice if you tapped your left or right knee more frequently, or if your thoughts were distributed relatively evenly between past and future thoughts. This practice illuminates how rarely you simply rest in the awareness of the present moment and how often thoughts of the past or future dominate your current reality. If you've noticed this for yourself, don't worry! Simply noticing this habit is a great place to start building awareness.

If you think about it, much of the unhappiness or discontent you feel within your relationship to food and your body stems from this lack of being present in the here and now. Many of the examples presented at the beginning of this chapter reflect this theme. Some other examples may include:

✔ **A constant focus on a future point in time:** Many people are constantly thinking about losing weight or thinking about a food they want to eat. This places a strong emphasis on thinking about the future and what they believe it will be like when they get there. Many people even forfeit their own happiness in the present because they think they'll be happier after they get to this more desirous point in time.

✔ **A constant dwelling in the past:** Many people who struggle with their food and eating habits can also get caught up with past actions and find it hard to let go if they feel they slipped up and ate something they shouldn't have. This makes it challenging to focus on the present and all that the now moment has to offer.

Wanting your future to be different than the present moment is okay and can be a powerful motivator for change. But this motivation for change must be rooted in acceptance of the present moment, not from trying to solve your problems. Mindfulness emphasizes acceptance first, and from there change may or may not occur. This acceptance is not passive by any means, it's simply resting with what is in the present moment and from there making a conscious decision as to whether you want to continue recreating that reality for yourself or not. All your now moments do indeed influence and affect the future moments of your life.

Now that you've explored and been introduced to both mindful eating and mindfulness, you've laid the first stepping-stone on your path towards a healthier, more mindful you. You've also set a solid foundation upon which you can now build as you explore the rest of this book and all that mindful eating has to offer you.

Chapter 2

What You Can Expect to Gain (or Lose) from Mindful Eating

I'm not going to try to convince you that mindful eating is another magic bullet to weight loss or that within seven days you'll never want to overeat or experience another food craving ever again. Eating mindfully is not a quick-fix approach to your food-related woes, but it is a long-term solution that offers countless rewards and will benefit you in ways that you've never thought possible.

In this chapter I'll explore some of these benefits and how mindful eating can help contribute to a healthier, happier life.

The Benefits of Mindfulness

Mindful eating is simply an extension of applying the power of mindfulness to everyday living, so exploring some of the benefits of mindfulness in general is a good place to start. The benefits of mindfulness are nothing to scoff at – the following list is proven, powerful and profound! Mindfulness as a practice has been shown to help people:

- ✔ Decrease anxiety
- ✔ Reduce fatigue
- ✔ Decrease depression
- ✔ Improve focus and attention
- ✔ Stabilize moods and reduce mood disturbances
- ✔ Improve emotional resiliency
- ✔ Improve self-awareness
- ✔ Aid with stress management
- ✔ Improve self-esteem
- ✔ Improve perception of body image
- ✔ Decrease the experience of physical pain
- ✔ Decrease blood pressure
- ✔ Slow heart rate
- ✔ Improve ability to relax
- ✔ Strengthen the immune system

No wonder mindfulness is no passing fad! More and more people are reaping the benefits of mindfulness and using it as a tool to help discover a richer relationship with life, and that includes a healthier relationship with food.

The Rewards of Mindful Eating

Reading through the previous list of mindfulness benefits, you can see how this ancient practice can lend you a helping hand when it comes to your relationship with food. How often do you turn to food when you're feeling tired, stressed, anxious, lonely, over-emotional, sad or depressed, or because of low self-esteem or poor body image? Or rush through eating something without paying attention? These key benefits can most certainly help you find a more balanced approach to eating and relating to food.

More specifically, on top of all those wonderful mindfulness benefits, a few additional rewards of mindful eating include helping you to:

✔ Cope with disordered eating

✔ Regulate eating habits

✔ Modify or change eating behaviors

✔ Work with impulse control

✔ Reduce binge-eating episodes

✔ Manage weight effectively

Don't you just love how one simple act can lead to a whole ripple effect of more positive benefits? I like to call this the *up-spiral*. So many more rewards ripple out to affect all areas of your life – like improving your relationships with other people, improving your work life and your spiritual life. These kinds of benefits – truly feeling amazing in your body, mind and spirit – are the deeper reasons that you're embarking on this mindful eating journey.

If you've struggled with food in one way or another, some of these benefits may strike a chord. Whether you're struggling with losing weight, suffering with a disease like diabetes, trying to change unhealthy eating patterns to healthier ones, have been caught in a cycle of binging, or are suffering from impulsive or mindless eating, then mindfulness can help you to carve out a new path and offers you truly profound benefits that may include:

✔ Finding a healthy balance within your relationship with food.

✔ Discovering peace of mind.

✔ Reconnecting with nature and your food source.

✔ Feeling good in your body, mind and spirit.

✔ Feeling a sense of happiness, meaning and purpose in life.

Underneath the more superficial changes that we all seek and strive to make lies a fundamental and human desire to feel in balance, peaceful, content, healthy, happy and, ultimately, fulfilled in our lives.

In your mindful eating journal (flip to Chapter 4 for more on starting a mindful eating journal) write down your top three initial benefits that you hope to gain through mindful eating.

Now look at this list. What intentions or motivations lie underneath your desire to achieve these benefits? What are the deeper, more meaningful benefits that you're looking to align with?

The next section looks at some of the fruitful benefits of beginning to eat more mindfully.

Feeling good in your body

One of the main reasons that people turn towards pursuing a healthier lifestyle (whether they do this in healthy or unhealthy ways) is because they want to feel better in their bodies. The good news is that mindful eating can help you to feel great in your body. Doesn't that sound nice? The desire to feel good in your body naturally stems from a desire to experience happiness in your life, because having a more enjoyable experience in your body contributes to a more enjoyable life experience. Would you say this is true for you?

Some people are so hooked on trying to achieve optimal health that the effort causes them to be unhappy! Achieving health requires a balanced and holistic lifestyle approach to health and wellbeing.

Grab your mindful eating journal and a pen and explore the following questions: what does 'feeling good in your body' mean to you? Feeling good in your body may mean feeling at ease, feeling peaceful, content, joyful, healthy, strong, flexible, rested, energetic, relaxed and so on.

What is the result or benefit of feeling this way? How do you know when you feel good in your body? When was the last time you felt good in your body? On a scale of one to ten (ten being the best) how good do you feel in your body right now?

Mindful eating helps you feel good in your body for a number of reasons. Before examining some of those reasons, take a look at why your relationship to food may be preventing you from feeling what you deserve – absolutely amazing.

Feeling subpar?

As I've discovered over years of working with mindful eating clients, many people don't initially make the connection that the way they're choosing to eat (or mindlessly engaging with food) is contributing to a feeling of dis-ease or discontent, preventing them from feeling good not only in their bodies, but also causing them dissatisfaction and unhappiness in their lives.

The way you relate to food (if you relate in a mindless manner) may be causing you to feel discontent in your body for a number of reasons:

- ✔ You're not paying attention to the association between eating certain foods and physical pain or discomfort, like a sore stomach, headaches, inflammation, indigestion, congestion, constipation, acid reflux, allergic reactions and similar ailments.

- ✔ Mindlessly eating without consciously choosing what kind of food you're eating is contributing to weight gain or disease.

- ✔ You're not paying attention to the amount of food that you're eating and excess calories are contributing to weight gain and general discomfort in your body.

- ✔ Mindlessly munching and eating despite a lack of hunger, including eating as a way to distract, avoid, procrastinate, soothe emotions and reduce stress, may be causing discomfort and discontent.

- ✔ Getting caught up in a cycle of craving and addiction where your attention is focused on pursuing the food of your desire despite thoughts like, 'I shouldn't eat that' is causing you more suffering than you perhaps realize.

Mindful eating helps you to become aware of the many aspects of your eating, including what you're eating, how you're choosing to eat, why you're choosing to eat it and how your food choices are making you feel. You also become aware of your thoughts surrounding food and how your thinking mind is affecting and influencing your food choices.

Think back to the last time you overstuffed yourself. Close your eyes and imagine yourself right back in that situation.

Maybe you were home alone watching a movie, out for dinner with friends or over at your aunt's house for a family holiday gathering. In your mindful eating journal describe how you felt. Would you say you were uncomfortably full? Were you so full it hurt? Did you feel sluggish or lethargic, or suffer from low energy after you ate? Or did overeating make you jump for joy? Overall, did you feel better or worse after you mindlessly overate?

If you're like most people, you classified your last overeating experience as less than enjoyable; mindlessly overeating doesn't usually feel good. It doesn't bring you the lasting happiness that you're truly yearning for, but rather a more immediate feeling of discomfort and pain that is both physical and oftentimes emotional.

Mindfully Moving towards Feeling Better about Your Body

Becoming more mindful of your eating experience allows you to feel good in your body because it encourages you to:

✔ **Listen to what your body is communicating to you.** As a result, your body is fed the appropriate amount of food, preventing needless overeating.

✔ **Reduce your brain fog.** What and how you eat can contribute to mental sluggishness. Are you familiar with overeating-induced brain fog? Eating the right amount for your body helps improve your mental capacities and helps you to stay mentally clear, sharp and focused throughout your day.

✔ **Eat the right amount and not overeat (or under-eat).** Eating the right amount of food results in brighter moods and more stable energy levels.

In addition to these three benefits, there are four more primary reasons why mindful eating helps you to feel good in your body:

✔ It helps you to break free from chronic dieting.

✔ You can regulate weight levels with a holistic lifestyle approach.

✔ You can reduce and manage stress.

✔ You can prevent and manage chronic diseases.

Breaking free from dieting

Dozens – no, hundreds – of diets are out there, all competing for your attention and, more importantly, your money. The dieting industry is a multi-billion-dollar industry, and yes, that was billion with a *B!* Many diets proclaim that you can 'lose ten pounds in ten days', lose belly fat, slim down, tone up and look years younger.

Most diets, within our current cultural definition of them, don't work. Some of the reasons they don't work are because most diets:

✔ Are too extreme.

✔ Are too rigid.

✔ Focus on deprivation and starvation.

✔ Suck all the pleasure out of eating.

✔ Don't address your underlying relationship with food and eating and why you may habitually tend to over-eat, return to unhealthy foods or use food as a coping mechanism.

The other two reasons aren't so much to do with the diets, but rather the way most people approach them:

✔ People tend to set unrealistically high expectations for their new diets.

✔ People tend to want unrealistically fast results from the diet.

Open your mindful eating journal and make a list of how many diets you've been on. Now think about the last diet you went on. What was that experience like for you? Did you lose weight on that diet? What happened when you went off the diet? Did you gain the weight back?

Because many people do initially lose weight on a restrictive diet, people commonly associate that initial weight loss with the positive results of the diet. But weight *regain* is a reality for a large majority of all dieters! Most people blame themselves and their lack of willpower for not being able to maintain the rigidity of the diet and extreme calorie restriction, but these approaches are not realistic or sustainable.

If you've tried countless different diets but have always found yourself right back where you started, you may find that one of the best benefits of eating more mindfully is that it offers you an opportunity to step out of a rigid diet mentality and into a balanced lifestyle mentality.

Most diets don't provide you with the long-term solution that you're seeking and can cause wild swings between allowing and restricting certain foods, fostering that all too familiar all-or-nothing mentality. Mindful eating offers you a middle-way path, allowing you to discover what your body really needs in each and every new moment.

Mindful eating is not another diet! This book contains no menu planning, and I'm not going to tell you what foods you should or shouldn't eat. Mindful eating is about developing and cultivating a healthy relationship with food – real food – that includes changing your attitudes about food, your body, your weight and your life.

Mindful eating doesn't advocate any particular dietary lifestyle; however, after you start to eat more mindfully, you may notice yourself gravitating towards healthier food choices, including whole, fresh and organic foods, which are discussed in Chapter 6.

Mindful eating helps you to step out of the dietary box that you may be accustomed to putting yourself in. A dietary box tends to be rigid and doesn't leave the door open for you to really listen to your body and what it's communicating to you. Rigidly defined dietary boxes tend to favor the thinking mind over the feeling body and tend to separate you further from your capacity to eat intuitively.

Following a dietary framework (like vegetarianism or veganism) as a lifestyle approach can definitely be beneficial, but give yourself permission to invite in your awareness and move freely using your intuition.

Dietary boxes tend to set the bar extremely high, perpetuating cycles of an all-or-nothing mentality where you're either 'on the wagon' or 'off the wagon', which sets you up for self-critical thoughts, guilt, shame and blame.

Mindful eating releases the need for crash dieting (in the conventional sense of deprivation and restriction) and offers a more holistic, balanced lifestyle approach.

The term *balanced* as used here is not referring to a *balanced* diet, where you give yourself permission to eat healthy foods balanced with junk foods, for example (although you may choose to). *Balanced* in this sense points to internal balance, where you experience freedom from the food struggle and feel happy and content in your life. You can decide which dietary approach aligns with and matches this internal balance.

Remember that your body is literally changing on a daily, weekly and monthly basis. Your body changes through the seasons, as you age and as you go through different experiences like pregnancy or illness. A more flexible way of approaching your relationship with food is to listen to what your body is communicating to you. You do this by becoming aware, practicing mindfulness and incorporating many of the tools and mindful eating skills offered throughout this book.

Shedding the excess: losing weight

Everyone wants to know the secrets to weight loss – well, guess what? Mindfulness is one of those secrets. But it's a secret that's perhaps too well kept and often overlooked – at least initially. After years of yo-yo dieting and repeated failed weight-loss attempts people seem to be more inclined to give mindful eating a fair chance. I wonder why? Most people prefer to opt for quick-fix approaches, but they usually find themselves right back where they started.

Although mindful eating is by no means a quick-fix solution, you can start to see results as soon as you start implementing mindfulness in the moments of your life. Mindful eating is a long-term approach to weight-loss that's worth all the time you're willing to dedicate to it.

Mindful eating does not have to be a stand-alone approach to weight loss; you can combine it with any other efforts you're making for added benefits. For example, if you're following a particular dietary lifestyle like the raw food lifestyle, vegetarianism or veganism, combine and integrate mindful eating into your eating routine. Mindful eating doesn't advocate a specific dietary approach: remember, it's about how you eat, the way you eat and why you eat, although it can help guide you to healthier food choices (flip to Chapter 6 for more on choosing healthy food).

Mindful eating is an inside-out approach to weight loss because you're intuitively making decisions about what and how much to eat based on becoming aware of what your body is communicating to you. Here are some of the reasons why mindfulness can help prevent weight gain and allow you to maintain your optimal weight:

✔ Mindful eating helps you clue into hunger and fullness signals from your body, helping you stop eating when you've had enough and allowing you to notice how often you're eating when you're not hungry. Check out Chapter 8 for more on tuning in with the hunger-fullness scale.

✔ When you apply mindfulness to your eating process, you're more likely to notice triggers that cue you to eat when you are and aren't hungry. Chapter 3 contains more on food triggers.

✔ Mindfulness prevents excessive snacking and mindless munching by eating without distractions. Look at Chapter 8 for more on how to only eat when you eat.

When you implement some of the simple yet effective mindful eating techniques offered throughout this book, you may start to notice how much you've been eating unnecessarily. This reaction is quite common from newcomers to mindful eating and is exactly the kind of information that your body has been trying to communicate to you. But now, you're paying attention, listening and taking action to live in alignment with your body's messages.

Time out: reducing stress

If I asked you to simply stand up, both feet on the floor and just stand there, would you consider that stressful? Okay, not exactly. But what if I asked you to stand for five hours? Or better yet, for a full day with no pee breaks and no sleep, or for a full month? What if, while you were standing there for the next five hours, full day or whole month, I asked you to stand on one foot and then balance an egg on a spoon? Stress is like that. One thing on its own is not necessarily stressful, but stress can slowly build up over time. The daily to-do list gets longer, and at the same time you're trying to earn a decent living. You discover more commitments and more expectations for you to succeed. All of these demands keep piling up along with the food on your plate. Could there be a connection? At least for some of us, there is.

Do you notice that when you experience higher stress levels, you also have a tendency to make poor food choices?

If you do, you're not alone. Stress makes it more challenging to bolster up willpower and resist giving in to poor food choices. In other words, stress makes it harder to say no and easier to say yes in the face of unhealthy foods. That's because stress activates the part of the brain that has impulsivity written all over it, and effectively shuts the lights out in the part of the brain that saves you from yourself with willpower and self-control. When you feel stressed, thoughts of 'I want to be the healthiest I can be' go flying out the window, and instead you mindlessly reach for habitual patterns you'd rather leave behind but that you're still carrying around, like a deadweight around your ankle.

Managing stress is one of the most important things that you can do for yourself in today's fast-paced lifestyle. When stress runs rampant like a wild elephant in your life, it prevents you from doing the things that help manage stress in the first place. Stress makes it harder to sit quietly alone in daily meditation, and it makes it more challenging (but not impossible) to get outside and go for that walk or run. Stress stops you from making your lunch the night before so that you don't eat out at that restaurant that you know doesn't have great food options. Basically, when stress gets out of control, self-care plummets, mostly because you think that you don't have time. But if you're familiar with these stress-induced experiences, you may realize that you can't afford *not* to take the time to care for yourself and manage stress more effectively.

You can use the practice of mindfulness as an integrated approach to effective stress management and thereby take a holistic approach to health and wellness. A holistic approach is not just about what you do or don't eat, it's also about how you manage stress, in addition to how well you sleep at night, how much playtime you get in your life and how much sunshine you get (the list goes on) that determines the totality of your health and how you feel.

Mindful eating is one of the mindfulness practices that you can use in your daily life to help you manage stress. Sitting down to a meal, focusing on your senses and pausing to take a few deep breaths may sound simple – and it is – but it also has the power to help you manage and cope with the everyday stressors of your life, which can benefit you in innumerable ways.

Managing chronic health conditions

Mindfulness can also help you cope with and manage chronic health conditions, directly, or as an added bonus of effectively managing stress. Here are a few examples:

Improving digestion

Did you know that digestion actually starts in your mouth? When you gulp down large bites of food, you put added strain on your digestion as it has to process and break down the large morsels of food. Incorporating mindful eating techniques like slowing down and chewing your food more thoroughly takes some of the pressure off your gut to do all the work digesting the food, and you more thoroughly enjoy and taste your food!

Gastrointestinal disorders

Mindful eating may also help people with more serious digestive or gastrointestinal disorders. The perception of stress plays a key role in gastrointestinal disorders like irritable bowel syndrome (IBS), because stress has a very real physical effect on the body, and in this case, stress can stimulate colon spasms in people with IBS. Results show that participants of the Mindfulness-based Stress Reduction program (MBSR) experienced an improvement in their IBS-related quality of life.

Binge Eating Disorder

Mindful eating is now recognized to help people struggling with binge eating disorder (BED), which is characterized by eating large amounts of food without subsequent purging. Thanks to the work of Jean Kristeller, who developed the Mindfulness-based Eating Awareness (MB-EAT) program, countless individuals who suffer from BED are reducing binge-episode days per month as well as reducing depression through the application of mindfulness and mindful eating.

Type II diabetes

Being overweight raises your risk for type II diabetes. Using mindful eating as a way to manage weight can therefore also help this disease. (There's that up-spiral again!) Stress can also affect blood glucose levels, a primary concern for people living with diabetes. The stress hormone cortisol, when consistently elevated over time, continuously produces glucose, which leads to chronically elevated blood sugar levels. The good news is that implementing mindful eating techniques and incorporating mindfulness into your daily life can help you manage stress and prevent the consequences of weight gain and elevated blood glucose levels.

According to a study published in *Clinical Nutrition*, people with type II diabetes were more likely to be fast eaters than people without diabetes. Mindful eating can help you to slow down and chew your food more thoroughly.

The MB-EAT program has also been adapted for people with diabetes (called MB-EAT-*D*) where the participants are encouraged to combine inner wisdom and mindful self-awareness with outer wisdom, which includes knowledge about nutrition and concerns related to diabetes. The program has been shown to help improve weight loss and glycemic control amongst people with type II diabetes.

Feeling Good in Your Life

As I've already alluded to, the juiciest reward of all the combined benefits of mindful eating discussed so far is the gift of increased happiness, joy and contentment in your life. Sounds wonderful, doesn't it?

Whether you're consciously aware of it or not, most of your day-to-day decisions stem from the underlying motivation of the pursuit of happiness. When it comes down to it, most people simply want to be happy. Isn't this what most people are striving for in life? You work long hours to earn an income, spend time at the gym, get married, buy a house, have children, eat low-fat salad dressing – you do all of these things, ultimately, because you think they'll bring you a greater sense of happiness. Even if you want a sense of security or seek success or are searching for greater balance or fulfillment, you usually want these things because you think they'll bring you happiness.

Minding Happiness

All the benefits and rewards of mindful eating listed in this chapter ultimately point towards this primary benefit of happiness. Paying attention while eating may encourage you to eat less, which may result in the benefit of weight loss, which then may prevent obesity-related diseases like type II diabetes. Tuning into your body allows you to listen carefully to what your body is communicating to you, and as a result you feel great in your body, which allows you to feel a sense of peace in your mind, and naturally brings greater happiness in your life. Everything comes into harmonious alignment – body, mind and spirit.

Some of the ways mindful eating lends itself to increased happiness are because mindfulness helps you:

- Become more satisfied with less.
- Have the freedom to make conscious choices.

✔ Free yourself from the struggle with food.

✔ Gain greater enjoyment from food and eating.

✔ Step out of the vise-like grip of a dieting mentality and into a lifestyle-oriented approach to health and wellbeing.

✔ Truly appreciate the miracle of your body, your life and the food that enables you to live the life of your choosing.

Like most people, if you dig deep into your relationship with food and look at your underlying motivations surrounding the food-related decisions you make, you'll find that you simply want to feel good in your body, feel at peace in your mind and feel a sense of happiness in your life.

Discovering true contentment

One of the greatest gifts that mindfulness offers you is the ability to discover joy, peace, contentment and happiness in the present moment. I call this the primary, or fundamental, benefit of mindfulness because it's what everyone seeks in life. Mindfulness can serve it up to you on a silver platter, right here, right now, without you having to struggle to get there – happiness is already here waiting for you to experience it.

In pursuit of happiness

Happiness is a tricky topic to cover, and it's usually not what you think it is – some ideal, imagined future point in time.

Happiness is somewhat of a paradox. As soon as you try to pursue your idea of happiness – perhaps you become fixated on the idea that being ten pounds lighter will make you happier in your life – then happiness, which only lives in the present moment, slips through your fingers because you've become hyper-focused on getting to that happier place at a future point in time.

The practice of mindfulness welcomes in true contentment through witnessing the present moment without judgment – not an easy task! As soon as you start getting ideas and thinking about what happiness is and what you have to do to get it, you've lost it! The present moment is the only place where true happiness lives, not at that magical place where you're ten pounds lighter, have a new tint in your hair or have managed to make it through two weeks of a restrictive diet.

On the other hand (and this is the paradoxical part), the actions that you take in the now moments of your life (whether you choose the salad or the hamburger) influences how you experience the future moments of your life. So you can lose weight and feel happiness as a result, but as soon as you pursue weight-loss because you think it will bring greater happiness, you've embarked on a losing battle.

Staying present is a key ingredient to feeling a sense of fundamental joy and happiness in your life, and that's what mindful eating encourages you to do – take mindful bites in the present moment, feel fulfilled and nourished by food and by life, and make conscious, health-supporting choices now, which also set the stage for enjoyable future present-moments as well.

You ultimately have the power to feel joy and happiness in each and every moment, no matter what your circumstances are or how much you weigh or what disease you're struggling with. Some may say feeling thrilled about life is more challenging when you feel overweight, unhealthy, diseased or gripped by cravings and food addiction. Taking care of your body and being mindful of your eating habits is what supports you in living a happy life, and, in many ways, health lends itself to happiness.

Freedom from the Struggle

When you confuse pleasure with happiness, suffering can result. Oftentimes you seek out food because you think it offers you happiness – or at least a moment of bliss within your busy life. But that pleasurable sense of happiness is only fleeting and impermanent, and you can become hooked on constantly trying to recreate the pleasure that you seek to hold onto, resulting in a more challenging relationship with food.

If you've ever struggled with food in the past, or perhaps still do, then you know all too well that when you get caught in this struggle with food and eating, it can cause you a lot of emotional pain and hardship. This pain can be frustrating to experience because a lot of the time you feel that you should be the one in control of food, not the other way around.

Like working with any kind of addiction or trying to change any kind of habit, when you find yourself caught in an unhealthy cycle that is challenging to change, it can be all-consuming and tends to permeate and influence the other areas of your life as well. It can affect your relationships with your friends and loved ones, it can influence the decisions you make and the opportunities you choose to take (or pass up), and it can also influence your family and work life.

Mindfulness can help end the struggle with food, and in fact, it's an essential component in helping you to do so! Mindful eating allows you to see how your relationship with food is affecting the days, months and years of your life and offers you a way to connect with a deeper sense of happiness, purpose and life fulfillment.

Ironically, as a human being you tend to seek happiness in immediate pleasure (insert your addictive tendencies here: TV, shopping, gambling, drinking, eating and so on), which usually results in pain and suffering. You think that chocolate cake makes you happy, when although it may bring about a moment of pleasure, it may also add to your life-long battle with excess weight and all the suffering and unhappiness that goes along with that.

Have you ever felt gripped by a food craving so strong that you felt like you had no choice but to give in? Perhaps you felt helpless and that you had no other option but to succumb to the intensity of the urge, regardless of any consequences. This feeling is quite common amongst people who struggle with food.

The good news is that mindfulness dishes up a generous serving of freedom – the freedom to choose and the freedom to say no when your mind is craving, yet your body is not hungry. Mindful eating gives you the ability to say yes or no and to choose how much, what and when you want to eat. Mindful eating puts you in the driver's seat, and you get to decide how you want to navigate your mindful eating journey.

Part II
Preparing the Ground for Mindful Eating

Top five ways to start preparing for your mindful eating

✔ **Explore the flip-side to mindfulness:** by understanding how your mind is preoccupied with being everywhere else but right here, you can start catching your mindless moments and train your mind to be present with your experience.

✔ **Start noticing your triggers:** practice paying attention to what's triggering you to eat when you're not actually hungry. See if you can pay more attention to those triggers and how your knee-jerk-reactions are prompting you to act.

✔ **Set realistic expectations and identify your goals:** understand how mindfulness can help you reach your health goals and write down what goals you'd like to achieve.

✔ **Cultivate a supportive attitude that fosters mindfulness:** examine some of these attitudes, including acceptance, non-judgment, curiosity and self-compassion.

✔ **Practice mindfulness while choosing what to eat and during meal preparation:** mindfulness isn't only about paying attention while you eat, it can also help you decide what to eat and help you to stay present while you're making those foods into a delicious meal.

Get more information on recognizing the characteristics between mindfulness and mindlessness and how to apply them to eating mindfully at www.dummies.com/extras/mindfuleating.

In this part . . .

- ✔ You have the opportunity to build a solid foundation by understanding the flipside to the mindful eating coin: *mindlessness*.
  You discover why you're geared towards automatic pilot and
  the difference between mindfulness and mindlessness.

- ✔ Explore how to find a middle-way approach to eating and how
  to achieve your health goals with mindful eating.

- ✔ Find out how to cultivate a supportive mindful eating mindset and
  how to grow the right attitudes to help you on this journey.

- ✔ Discover how to choose foods more mindfully and apply the
  power of mindfulness to the preparation of meals.

Chapter 3

Getting Mindless by the Mouthful

*I*f you're reading this book, chances are you've struggled with mindless eating in one form or another. Don't worry, you're not alone. In fact, everyone experiences mindlessness on a daily, even hourly, basis. As I explore in this chapter, everyone is geared towards mindlessness to a certain degree. Mindlessness isn't inherently a bad thing and can actually serve some important functions in your life. But if you don't start paying attention to how often you're not paying attention, mindlessness starts to dominate your life – and your eating habits.

Mindfulness versus Mindlessness

In order to fully understand mindfulness you also need to explore its flip side, *mindlessness* – something I'm sure you're familiar with.

Think of mindfulness and mindlessness as two sides of the same coin. Whichever one you choose to focus on is the one you naturally foster and strengthen.

But what's the difference between the two?

Mind-less-ness: Less of what?

The word *mindlessness* confuses some people. I've heard many people say that at first they thought mindlessness meant 'not thinking', because they thought the *less* in mindlessness implies 'less thinking'.

Actually, mindlessness means the complete opposite. Mindlessness indicates a wandering mind: thinking about anything other than what you're currently doing.

Mindlessness implies *more* thinking and *less* direct experiencing.

What's your frame of mind?

The table below is a quick guide to the differing characteristics of mindlessness and mindfulness. Keep in mind that these are generalizations – exceptions do exist! (Trick question: Can a person act out a habitual routine in a mindful way?)

Mindlessness	Mindfulness
Inflexible, rigid	Flexible
Unintentional	Intentional
Reactive	Responsive
Automatic	Deliberate
Minimal information processing	Increased information processing
Passive, reduced attention	Engaged and active attention
Dull	Alert
Deliberate	Controlled
Routine	Variable
Wandering mind	Focused mind

Mind-full-ness: Full of what?

On the other hand, when you look at the word *mindfulness* you could mistakenly assume that the mind is *full*. And what is the mind usually full of? You guessed it: thoughts. Yet mindfulness actually implies awareness rather than thinking, as described in Chapter 1. When you're mindful, you observe your thoughts, yet you're not attached to them or swept up by them. Instead, you're focused on what you're experiencing, through your senses and bodily sensations.

When you're mindful, you're *full* of direct experience in the present moment and *less* distracted by thinking.

Away with the fairies: Discovering the different forms of mindlessness

Mindlessness expresses itself in many different ways in your life. Any of the following situations is a form of mindlessness:

Mind-wandering, daydreaming and lost in thought

As you read these pages, you may notice your mind periodically wandering, and then coming back to the page, even though your eyes are diligently following along each line. Don't worry, I won't take it personally! It's less an indication of the quality of the material than of what it means to be human.

Absentmindedness and forgetfulness

Have you ever walked into a room for something and forgotten what it was you were going to get? Have you ever left the house wondering if you locked the door or left the stove on? These situations probably happen to you more often than you'd like.

Time travel

Spending time lost in thought worrying about your future or dwelling on the past is a normal tendency. If you're trying to lose weight, your thoughts constantly go to the future – 'when I lose these ten pounds . . . ' or the past – 'I can't believe I ate that this morning!' Another form mindlessness takes is when you're in a rush and your mind is constantly ten steps ahead of yourself.

Disregarding the consequences

Mindlessness also plays a role when you choose to ignore the consequences of decisions. I explore this aspect of mindfulness – awareness of food choices – in Chapter 6.

Rigid rules

Mindlessness means being caught in a rigid mindset and way of thinking and ignoring the greater contextual framework or other perspectives. You may accept your thoughts at face value, such as your beliefs – true or not – about food. Many of the decisions you make related to food and eating are unconscious, largely based on these belief systems.

When you're mindful you become more sensitive to the uniqueness of each situation; you can choose to make new choices without having to follow rigid rules that may not be appropriate to the situation. In this way, you give yourself the flexibility to decide what the best course of action is for *you*, instead of letting your actions be dictated and governed by rules.

Mindlessness for peak performance

Mindlessness can definitely come in handy, especially when it comes to honing advanced skills, such as those used by professional athletes. Think about basketball players. Over the years, they continuously practice perfecting the skill of throwing the basketball and getting it into the hoop. Over time this skill becomes mindlessly automatic; the way they hold the ball in their hands, the way they place their feet and jump as they shoot. This automatic behavior then allows them to become aware of and pay attention to other important aspects of the game, such as where other players are standing, who's moving where, how much time is left in the game, and so on.

Mindlessness isn't always necessarily a bad thing; use it to your advantage and make sure that you're conscious of what you tend to be unconscious of!

Mindless emotional reactions

In the same way that a skill or action can become mindlessly repetitive, so too can any emotional response. You mindlessly overreact rather than respond appropriately to a situation, habitually judge your experiences, feel self-critical, feel guilty or blame yourself for something that you did. You can also fall into the cycle of mindlessly resisting what you're feeling by using something like food as a method of distraction or becoming fixated on wanting or craving.

Look at the types of mindlessness discussed above and reflect on the last time you experienced any one of these mindless behaviors. Was it in the last day? The last hour? Or even the last few minutes?

When you're mindless you're more likely to be unaware of the present moment and the richness of the experience it offers you – in a sense, you're out of touch with reality. One of the consequences of mindlessness is that you become disconnected from your body and what you're feeling. A helpful way to become more in tune with your body is to practice the body scan, outlined in Chapter 8.

A busy mind, an active brain

Neuroscientists have been studying the brain for many years. In some studies, participants take part in activities like watching a scene unfold on a screen or solving math problems. Using technology like MRI scanners, researchers can see that the brain is highly active when it's engaged. This then begs the question, when it's not engaged, is the brain inactive?

Neuroscientists have set out to explore this question and learn what level of brain activity takes place when participants are asked to do nothing; to *not* focus or pay attention to anything in particular, but simply rest in a wakeful state. Although much of this research is still in its infancy, it seems that during non-engaged resting, the mind isn't actually resting at all but is surprisingly busy, wandering off in all sorts of directions!

Take a moment to put down this book and rest your mind. No need to focus on anything in particular. What do you notice? Where does your mind go? What kinds of thoughts arise for you? Did you lose yourself in thought at all?

Geared towards mindlessness

The brain seems to be somewhat geared towards mindlessness. Researchers now refer to this state as the *default state* or *default mode*, where a part of the brain called the default mode network (DMN) is activated. The mind tends to continuously revert to these wandering ways not only when we're in a resting state, but also about half the time when we're engaged in an activity! Everyone experiences this wandering mind from the task at hand; while driving, reading, watching TV, sitting in class, and of course, while eating.

The default mode is suspended during specific goal-oriented tasks where mindfulness, focus and attention are required, and then the brain reverts back to the default state when it is no longer focusing so intensely.

Mindlessly focused on self

The chronic mental chatter that goes on in the mind is associated with this default mode and tends to be introspectively self-focused, what neuroscientists refer to as *self-referential processing*. This means that whatever the mental chatter is about, whether you're ruminating about the future, dwelling on the past, criticizing or judging, thinking about or comparing yourself to other people, it's almost always concerned in some way with you and your sense of self.

Finding happiness through mindfulness

Ancient wisdom traditions claim that this state of mindlessness is one of the main sources of suffering and that you can actually experience a lot more joy and happiness in your life by disengaging the default state and activating mindful awareness in your life. The interesting part is that science is now backing up what the Buddhist tradition has been saying for many years. Research has shown that the state called *mind-wandering*, which can also be thought of as mindlessness, is associated with lower levels of happiness. In fact, one of the key signs of depression is a real difficulty in disengaging from this default state of mind-wandering.

Fortunately, mindfulness can retrain your mind to focus on the present moment instead of habitually falling into the default mode where it largely focuses on self-related thoughts. The default mode network in the brain has been shown to be less active in meditators than their non-meditating counterparts.

The amount of time spent lost in the default state of mind can indeed be a predictor of unhappiness, whereas present-moment awareness and mindfulness are good predictors of well-being and happiness.

Advantages of mindlessness

Mindlessness has both advantages and disadvantages; it's neither inherently good nor bad. Mindlessness evolved for good survival-based reasons, and being completely aware of each and every moment in an intentional and mindful way is almost impossible; in some cultures, this is the definition of attaining pure enlightenment!

Efficiently mindless

Mindlessness can and does play an important part in your life, and primarily it has to do with efficiency.

Everything you do with your brain, from thinking to decision making, requires a lot of energy. As a way to become more efficient, the brain is designed to streamline some of that activity in order to avoid over-expending energy. As I explained earlier, the unconscious part of the mind that runs on automatic pilot allows you to efficiently undertake skills and habits – which can be positive or negative.

Whenever it can, your brain encourages automatic behavior so that it doesn't waste energy constantly thinking about or making decisions, especially around things that you've already done countless times. You make innumerable decisions every single day; thinking about each and every one of them would be exhausting, so these automatic functions have many advantages.

Survival of the thinkers

As humans have evolved, it's become increasingly beneficial to have brains that use their downtime to think about potential threats or challenges to survival. In this way the mind is always problem solving to increase its chance of survival.

Think of this downtime as like the idling of a car. When your mind is at rest it still has a baseline of activity so that when it needs to take off again, it's ready to go and can take off faster. Your brain uses this mental downtime to process and categorize information to make future decision making and information processing easier.

Learning new skills and automatic pilot

Mindlessness also plays a large role in maintaining skill sets after you've learned them. At first, when you're learning something new, you have to pay attention to what you're doing.

After you learn the skill, the brain creates neural pathways that allow you to repeat the behavior without having to think about it – at which point your actions becomes automatic. When something becomes second nature, you operate on automatic pilot.

Think about riding your bike – all the steps that you need to perform to successfully get on your bike and start riding it. If you had to literally think about all those steps every time you rode your bike, you'd find it a lot more difficult! After you learn how to ride a bike, you can easily hop on your bike while talking on the phone (not recommended!) or thinking about other things.

Mindlessness allows you to engage in and carry out highly complex tasks with minimal mental involvement after you learn a skill. The mind steps aside and simply lets cellular memory run the show.

Mindlessness is especially helpful when you perform advanced skills as it allows you to execute multiple tasks at the same time.

Disadvantages of mindlessness

Although mindlessness has its advantages, as I'm sure you guessed, it can also be a double-edged sword.

Constant problem solving in our mental downtime can actually be a major source of suffering. Since your mind is geared towards problem solving, it tends to always be looking for problems and ways of resolving them, rather than resting in the present moment and enjoying it for what it is.

Mindlessness isn't always helpful, especially if you let too much of your life be governed by automatic pilot, routinely going through the motions of your day without paying much attention. If you're going about most of your day unconsciously, then you're missing out on the precious moments of your life – and what is the point of a life like that?

One of the biggest disadvantages to mindlessness is that if you let it run rampant, it can be a destructive force, especially when it comes to mindless eating and your health.

You may be driving your car only to arrive at your destination without being fully present for the drive, which may be fuel-efficient for the brain, but is also highly dangerous!

Or you may be sitting and eating lunch, but your thoughts are focused on the presentation you have to give after lunch rather than on the food in front of you, which again, may be helpful, but is also potentially dangerous!

Mindless Eating and the Disappearing Food Act

Have you ever looked down at an empty plate and wondered, 'Where did all the food go?' This is a classic example of mindless eating – of not paying attention while you eat – and everyone's experienced it to one degree or another.

Imagine you're sitting in front of your computer or the television and your hand reaches for another chip or cracker only to realize that the bag is empty. Perhaps you were just preoccupied with thoughts about a relationship, work, school, or your daily to-do list. Or imagine you're at a business meeting over lunch, being swept away by an engaging conversation, and before you know it, you've eaten a whole plate of food without realizing it – or tasting it.

Mindlessness especially governs your habitual behaviors – all those actions that you perform day in and day out. Eating happens to fall into this category, so understandably mindless eating is quite a challenge for many people.

Even mindless eating is not always a bad thing. This automatic behavior can actually be quite helpful when eating – it's what prevents you from spilling tomato sauce on your white shirt while skillfully navigating a business lunch meeting with your boss!

Are you eating mindlessly?

According to Brian Wansink, author of the book *Mindless Eating: Why We Eat More Than We Think* (Hay House, 2011), we make over 200 food-related decisions each and every day, most of which we're unaware of. When asked, most people say they only make about 30 food-related decisions on any given day.

If you're unaware of the present moment while eating, you may have a dissatisfying relationship with food. You may be eating mindlessly if:

- ✔ You're too busy to sit down to eat.
- ✔ When you sit down to eat, you're only focused on what you need to do next.
- ✔ You think about what you want to eat next while you're currently eating.
- ✔ You often eat at your desk at work.
- ✔ You eat while driving.

✔ You don't put thought or consideration into your food choices.

✔ You often eat in front of the television.

✔ You usually couple other activities with eating.

✔ You disregard the consequences of your food choices.

Being aware of cues and triggers to eat

You're constantly being triggered to eat mindlessly. Something happens and then *boom!* – you find yourself standing in front of the fridge with the door open looking for something to eat or grazing on last night's leftovers. You're walking down the street and before you know it you're standing in line for a fresh cinnamon roll, or you catch yourself driving up to the takeout window without much recollection of what happened and how you got there.

A trigger is a cue or signal that prompts a habitual action. Most of the time you're unaware of the trigger that propelled you towards food, whether you're hungry or not. Finding out how to identify and become aware of your triggers is one of the ways that you discover how to eat more mindfully.

The two reasons why you eat

An infinite number of reasons why you turn to food exist, all of which can be grouped into two main categories:

1. Because you're hungry.

2. And because you're triggered.

The first category relates to physical hunger and the second category relates to everything else; a category with an infinite number of possible food and eating triggers.

I explore physical hunger in Chapter 8 through the use of the hunger-fullness scale. For now, I look at the second category: the many triggers that are unrelated to physical hunger.

Exploring food triggers

Can you think of some of the ways that you've been triggered to eat without being hungry? Look at the following list and consider whether you've ever been triggered by these cues:

- ✔ Sensory triggers
- ✔ External triggers
- ✔ Internal triggers

Sensory triggers

Sensory triggers are cues that come from your senses, stimulating you to eat. Humans evolved mechanisms to help spare them from famine and overcome times of food scarcity. Because of these survival-based traits, your senses provide you with powerful cues that prompt you to load up on calories, even if you're not hungry, as a way to store fat in case of a future famine. Chapter 9 contains more on mindful exploration of the senses.

- ✔ **The sight of food**: seeing an ad on TV, someone eating a donut in front of you in line, the sight of a candy bowl on a desk.

- ✔ **The smell of food**: the smell of muffins as you walk past a bakery, coffee in a coffee shop or popcorn at the movie theater.

- ✔ **The sound of food**: someone opening a can of soda, grilling food on a barbecue or describing last night's meal to you.

- ✔ **The taste of food**: tasting a bite of a cookie prompts you to want to eat the whole box.

- ✔ **The texture of food**: the way you feel food in your mouth can also trigger you to eat more. If your mouth is craving something crunchy, you may eat chips to satisfy that craving.

External triggers

External triggers happen around us in our environment. The sight, smell and sound of food can also be classified as an external trigger. Some others include:

✔ **The time of day**: eating lunch at noon, whether you're hungry or not.

✔ **Time of year**: special occasions like Christmas and Thanksgiving can be rife with food triggers.

✔ **Weather or temperature outside**: cold, rainy days prompt a desire or craving for a specific food, perhaps warm soup.

✔ **Social situations**: the sight of other people eating and enjoying food.

✔ **Serving sizes**: this includes the size of packages and containers that food comes in and the size of the plates or bowls that you eat out of.

✔ **Visual quantity of food**: how much food you have in your fridge, especially perishable food, may trigger you to eat more in order to prevent waste and spoilage. Portion sizes and how much food you have on your plate as well as how much food is on the dining table during a meal.

✔ **Variety of food**: situations like all-you-can-eat buffets, with an assortment of foods, usually trigger most people to eat more than usual.

Internal triggers

Internal triggers are unique to you. External triggers can influence anyone present, but no one else can really know the internal triggers that influence your eating behavior.

✔ **Emotions**: calming excited or anxious nerves or using food as a pick-me-up to improve sad or lonely feelings.

✔ **Stress**: relieving stress from work, home, family or relationships can trigger mindless or excessive eating.

✔ **Procrastination or avoidance**: eating to avoid or put off working or something pressing that you have to do.

✔ **Feeling bored**: eating to fill an empty space.

✔ **Feeling tired**: low energy can trigger unhealthy eating habits.

Identifying the mindless eater in you

Exploring your mindless eating tendencies helps you acknowledge where you're starting from and identify the areas for you to focus on.

Ask yourself the following questions and make a checkmark next to the ones that best describe you.

I am a:

✓ Mindless overeater

✓ Mindless under-eater

✓ Too-busy-multitasking mindless eater

✓ Late-night mindless eater

✓ Mindless picker or grazer

✓ Holiday and special-occasion mindless eater

✓ Social mindless eater

✓ Emotional mindless eater

✓ Stressed mindful eater

✓ Highly influenced-by-others mindless eater

✓ Restaurant mindless eater

✓ Family dinner mindless eater

✓ Movie theater mindless eater

✓ Nervous mindless eater

✓ Guilty mindless eater

✓ Eat-by-the-clock mindless eater

✓ 'I deserve a reward' mindless eater

✓ 'It's free, so I'll eat it' mindless eater

✓ 'I may never have the opportunity to taste this again' mindless eater

✓ Public mindless eater

- ✔ Occasional mindless eater
- ✔ Private or secretive mindless eater
- ✔ 'What the heck, I may as well' mindless eater

Exploring your mindless eating benefits

In your mindful eating journal, make two columns. (Flip to Chapter 4 for information on starting a mindful eating journal.) Entitle the first column PURPOSE and in that column identify ways *mindless* eating has helped or supported you and what purpose it's served for you. Has it perhaps brought you comfort, helped you save time, relieve stress or acted as a reward? Make a list of everything and anything that comes to mind in regard to mindless eating.

In the second column write REPLACEMENT. Next to each Purpose entry on the left, write what you can do as a replacement instead. So if you wrote 'comfort' think up some other things that you could do to help you feel comforted. Maybe you can take a bath, hang out with loved ones or call a friend on the phone – whatever feels right for you.

This practice is very helpful when it comes to changing habits. By thinking about what you can do instead of mindless eating, you're priming the conscious part of the brain that helps support the creation of new habits.

Exploring your mindless eating drawbacks

When you eat mindlessly, you're often not aware of how much food you take in. For instance, when multitasking, such as eating and surfing the web at the same time, your mind is unable to concentrate on both actions simultaneously and frantically switches from one task to the other.

Key hunger-fullness signals in your brain can get lost when you're trying to do too many things at once, so your brain may not receive important signals that help regulate how much you eat. As a result, you keep eating past fullness.

Now that you've explored all the ways that mindless eating has helped or supported you, consider some of the ways that it hasn't. In what ways has mindless eating brought suffering or unhappiness into your life?

Having a Full Belly but Wanting More

Because food is so tasty and delicious, you turn to food for enjoyment and pleasure. Have you ever noticed that when you weren't paying attention and missed the experience of eating, you felt dissatisfied? Even though you feel physically full, you notice a sense of *wanting* more, right after you've eaten something. You can be physically full but feel emotionally unsatisfied from your eating experience. The reason is because food gives you so much more than simple physical nourishment – you need to be mindfully present when receiving this nourishment. When you're being mindful of the eating experience, both the body and the mind are connected to the experience, allowing you to register a full experience, leaving you feeling contented and satisfied.

In our culture, a strong emphasis on reducing food to its nutritive properties exists – counting calories, grams of fat, milligrams of sodium and so on. Yet food does so much more than nourish our bodies physically; it nurtures us mentally, emotionally and even spiritually as well.

In your mindful eating journal note the last time you ate something and realized you barely experienced eating it. How did you feel when you realized you weren't paying attention? Did you notice yourself still wanting to eat more even though you were full?

Chapter 4

Getting Ready for Your Mindful Eating Journey

*Y*our brain is incredibly adaptable when it comes to learning new skills. It can override old, mindless habits and embrace new, mindful ways of living and eating that are more supportive of your health goals and well-being.

In this chapter I prepare you for the mindful changes to come, looking at how you can lay the groundwork for a successful journey from mindless to mindful eating.

Discovering Your Middle-Way Approach

Extremism. You may be very familiar with it. If so, you're not alone. Extremism is quite common in our culture as many people struggle with an all-or-nothing mentality. For instance, extremism in eating can result in yo-yo dieting, which is an unpleasant cycle to get caught in. This type of eating pattern leads to the familiar oscillations between:

✔ Striving and then flopping

✔ Starting and then stopping

✔ Getting on the wagon and falling off the wagon

✔ 'I can do it' versus 'I can't do it'

✔ 'I'm going on a diet' and 'I'm a failure at dieting'

This extreme way of thinking is quite an obstacle for many people to overcome on their mindful eating journey and may even prevent them from getting started altogether; sometimes this mentality rationalizes that: 'If I can't do it perfectly, I'm not even going to bother trying.'

If you identify with this common all-or-nothing mentality, then discovering how to find the middle way helps you to navigate your relationship with food and get started on this journey at a pace that feels comfortable for you.

The Goldilocks zone: Finding your 'just right' approach

As in the story of *Goldilocks and the Three Bears,* you want to find a dietary approach that is 'not too hot' or 'not too cold' but that is 'just right'. Avoid being too loose or too strict with yourself, but rather find a middle way that feels just right for you.

The middle way means embarking on your mindful eating journey with a non-extreme attitude and approach. If you've struggled with perfectionism then you also know that trying to be perfect when it comes to eating can be just as detrimental as eating with total lack of awareness. See the related sidebar, 'Orthorexia: the unhappy result of perfectionism' for more on where unchecked perfectionism can lead.

I'm sure you won't be surprised when I give you the heads up that following the mindful, middle-way path isn't a straight shot to your desired destination. You need to use your intuition and inner guidance as your compass, pointing towards

Orthorexia: the unhappy result of perfectionism

A newly recognized pattern of problem eating called orthorexia is considered to be an extreme preoccupation and obsession with eating healthy foods and avoiding those perceived to be unhealthy. Orthorexia is more focused on the quality of food rather than the quantity, as seen with other eating disorders like anorexia, bulimia and binge-eating disorders. This extreme fixation with healthy foods actually leads to an unhealthy condition and lifestyle.

Orthorexic individuals are less able to take part in normal everyday activities, seclude themselves more from others and exhibit self-punishing behavior if they slip up with their eating. According to the National Eating Disorder Association (NEDA), the underlying motivations that lead to orthorexia are a strong compulsion for complete control, creating an identity through food choices and the desire to be thin and improve self-esteem.

health and, perhaps more importantly, happiness. In this way you can constantly adjust your course as you fine-tune your approach and find out what works best for you.

You can expect to veer from the middle-way path many, many times. This behavior is perfectly normal and is just how you discover what works and what doesn't work for you. Your journey will be challenging at times as you start to find out what balance means to you. The more you embrace a middle-way approach, the more you reduce the wild and chaotic fluctuations that accompany the familiar extremist approach to diet.

Only you can decide what this middle-way approach feels and looks like for you. Ultimately your goal is to develop and cultivate a relationship with your food and eating that is healthy, fulfilling and positive. Use your unique middle-way approach as your guide to help you navigate your food choices.

Too loose versus too strict

If you try an approach that is too loose and you give in to less than healthy cravings every day, you soon discover that your body doesn't feel good eating unnecessary calories when you're not hungry, so you fail to find the healthy and happy relationship with food that you're ultimately seeking. The same is true on the other end of the spectrum if your approach is too strict and you constantly obsess and hyper-focus on every single thing that you eat. Neither approach supports a happy relationship with food.

If you're too loose:

- ✔ You constantly go with the flow and eat what everyone else is eating.
- ✔ You aren't making the most healthful choices for yourself.
- ✔ You make up excuses to eat whatever you want.
- ✔ You are constantly overindulging.

If you're too strict:

- ✔ You're very restrictive about what you choose to eat.
- ✔ You label most foods as good or bad.
- ✔ You follow strict rules about what you should or shouldn't eat.
- ✔ You manage cravings by being self-critical and overly strict.
- ✔ You're constantly on a diet.
- ✔ You obsess about food and weight.
- ✔ You are always counting the calories when you eat.
- ✔ Your periods of restriction tend to be followed by periods of extreme overindulgence.
- ✔ You may be depriving your body of nutrition.

Ask yourself if you're too loose or too strict with your dietary choices. Can you identify more strongly with one or the other, or do you notice a tendency to swing between one and then the other?

Explore ways that you can carve a middle-way path for yourself by using your mindful eating journal (see the section 'Starting a Mindful Eating Journal' later in this chapter). Can you think of a time when you felt really balanced within your relationship with food? What did that feel like? What were some of the factors that supported a balanced feeling around food and eating?

Always following one particular approach or applying strict rules is challenging over time. Each moment is a new moment, presenting new, unique circumstances. Finding a one-size-fits-all approach is impossible, which is why most diets don't work. This is the reason that makes mindfulness so universally applicable. Your best bet is to discover how to navigate each situation with fresh awareness, an open and curious mind, and a strong, open line of communication with your body.

The middle-way approach reflects that every circumstance is different and applies flexible decision making to suit the situation instead of setting unrealistically high and rigid expectations that just set you up to fail.

Starting a Mindful Eating Journal

In case you're cringing at the thought of meticulously writing down everything that you eat and monotonously counting all your calories, you can breathe a sigh of relief – that's not what keeping a mindful eating journal is all about.

I highly recommend buying a separate notebook or special journal for your mindful eating journal. As I'm sure you've already noticed, you'll be using it throughout this book as a tool for self-reflection and a place to answer and write down self-reflection exercises. Writing out your thoughts and seeing what words, ideas, thoughts and perceptions are staring back at you is quite eye-opening.

A mindful eating journal is not a place where you judge yourself harshly for what you ate or didn't eat, but a place where you reflect on how judging yourself makes you feel.

A mindful eating journal can:

✔ Be a supportive companion to you on this journey.

✔ Offer you a safe place to express yourself.

✔ Encourage mindfulness of behaviors, thoughts and feelings.

✔ Be a place for you to work through and process emotions.

Although it doesn't necessarily have to be a food diary, you can also use your mindful eating journal in this way if you choose to. If you're focusing on mindful eating as a weight management tool, consider incorporating this aspect into your daily journaling. Writing down your foods consumed each day for one week is a proven behavior modification tool because it encourages you to become aware of everything you're eating.

If writing down everything that you eat in a day makes you nervous or want to run away in the other direction, you can:

✔ Write about this in your mindful eating journal.

✔ Use your journal for other purposes.

✔ Try it for a day as an experiment to explore what exactly it triggers in you.

Using your mindful eating journal as a food diary may not be appropriate for you if you already obsess about what you eat, count calories or chronically weigh yourself.

Most importantly, a mindful eating journal can offer you a place to reflect on how you're feeling about what you're eating, but it can certainly be coupled with food data as well for powerful results.

Table 4-1 shows a sample worksheet that you can copy into your mindful eating journal. Alternatively, keep a binder for printouts of these worksheets to use daily for a set amount of time, or when you feel like you can use some directed focus.

Table 4-1	Mindful Eating Worksheet			
	Breakfast	**Lunch**	**Dinner**	**Snacks**
Time				
Tune in to hunger level	Before:	Before:	Before:	Before:
	During:	During:	During:	During:
	After:	After:	After:	After:
What are you feeling before you eat?				
Mood, thoughts, emotions, physical sensations				
What did you eat?				
Where did you eat?				
Were you eating with distractions?				
What are you feeling after you eat?				
Comments/additional notes				

The Four A's to Successful Change

We all have habits around food that we want to change. These habits may be a particular concern for you and one of the initial reasons you decided to pick up this book.

If you identify with many of the mindless habits outlined in Chapter 3 that relate to your health and eating, you're not alone. And if you're looking to make a change, then you're in the right place. Change can be difficult; if it wasn't, losing weight or breaking an unhealthy habit would be a cinch. Establishing lasting change is a struggle, especially when those changes sit at odds with the behaviors that you've been reinforcing for many years.

What does it take to make long-lasting, effective change in the direction of a healthier, more mindful you? Four essential steps to changing habits are key. I call them the four A's to successful change.

Awareness

The first of the four A's, awareness is an essential element in establishing an intentional change of habits. You can't make change happen without first becoming aware of what it is you want to change! Mindfulness is an indispensable tool in helping to cultivate awareness around your relationship with food.

How can you become aware of your unawareness? Many of the self-reflections and mindfulness practices in this book are good places to start. Have you ever experienced a sudden recognition that 'I just ate that without realizing it'? That's your awareness shining through! Awareness is when you catch yourself doing something, like the moment that you snapped back into reality after you caught yourself daydreaming.

Catching yourself acting in a mindless way means that you have just brought awareness to the situation. Way to go! Awareness is the first step towards change. Falling into the trap of putting yourself down when you do something you're not proud of or something you're feeling bad about is easy. But remember; at least now you're bringing awareness to the situation rather than letting your feelings continue to reside in the realm of the unconscious. Remind yourself that being aware is a very important and necessary step towards starting to eat more mindfully. This thought helps prevent you from feeling bad, which can trigger turning to more food to help you feel better, perpetuating an unhealthy eating cycle. Be patient with yourself, give yourself some credit and even congratulate yourself for shining the light of awareness on eating habits that are no longer serving you.

The path towards mindful eating takes time. Don't expect to be 100 per cent aware of everything you eat from now on – this expectation is not realistic. You're sure to find yourself in many more mindless eating situations somewhere along the road. This behavior is normal and to be expected.

When you do notice yourself eating mindlessly, open up your mindful eating journal and ask yourself the following questions with a self-compassionate and non-judgmental attitude (Chapter 5 delves into cultivating a supportive mindful eating mindset):

1. Why did I just eat mindlessly?

2. Can I think of a particular trigger that was involved?

3. Can I remember what I was feeling while I was eating?

4. Who else was involved? Was I alone or with other people?

5. What time of day was it?

6. Was I feeling tired, stressed or emotional beforehand?

7. How can I go about the situation differently next time to help me to eat more mindfully?

Acceptance

Acceptance is the second of the four A's. After you become aware of what you want to change, the next step is practicing acceptance (Chapter 5 explores acceptance more in depth). Acceptance is about acknowledging responsibility in a loving, self-compassionate way. It's recognizing that you've been reinforcing a mindless habit for perhaps a very long time and accepting where you are in the present moment. Through acceptance you acknowledge that the habits you've been strengthening are not contributing to your happiness and you consciously choose to make a change. This also means that if you want to make change happen, you need to accept what you have to do to make that change.

Acceptance is not resignation or giving up. It's quite the opposite. Acceptance is an inherent part of mindfulness that allows you to recognize habitual patterns with kindness and become self-aware, allowing you to make new choices for yourself.

Alignment

Alignment, number three of the four A's, kicks in after you've become aware of what you want to change and have fully accepted and embraced yourself and the situation in the present moment. You can then determine in which direction you'd rather be heading. Think of it as aligning your compass to match your desired destination.

In your mindful eating journal, consciously explore your vision of a healthy, mindful relationship with food. What does your mindful eating destination look like? What does it *feel* like for you to be eating more mindfully? Use as many *feeling* descriptors as possible. For example, 'I feel at peace, calm, nourished, grounded, grateful,' and so on.

Try to stay grounded, centered and rooted in the present moment during this visioning process so that you're not swept up by your thoughts of chasing or longing for a more desirable time in the future.

Action

When you've become aware, accepted and aligned with your new direction, the fourth A comes into play; it's time to take action to get there! Consider how committed you are to change and what specific actions you need to take to become a more mindful eater. You have to set goals, have realistic expectations and positive intentions, all of which I explore later in this chapter.

In order to successfully implement change, you need to be willing to take all four steps. Many people struggle with or get stuck at one or two (or even all!) of these steps.

In your mindful eating journal, write down which of these four steps you think you may struggle with. Which ones do you think you need support with? Are you aware that you struggle with mindless eating in front of the TV, but need an action plan to help you change this habit to become more mindful? Are you having a hard time with number two, accepting that mindless eating is not benefiting you, but is actually causing you a lot of pain and suffering?

Achieving Your Goals with Mindful Eating

If you're like most people, you're reading this book because you have in mind some desired outcome you'd like to see as a result of your mindful eating efforts. In this section, I look at establishing realistic expectations and non-striving goals to help you accomplish what you want to achieve.

Setting realistic expectations

Everyone has expectations – but are they really beneficial? The power of expectations can be huge; you can use them to help motivate yourself, but when misused, discouragement and disappointment can set in and totally set you up for failure.

Assessing expectations

Setting realistic expectations is a great place to start, and identifying attainable goals is important in setting a positive tone when establishing them. See the later section 'Identifying your health goals' for more.

In your mindful eating journal, make a list of some of your expectations of mindful eating. Look at your list and ask yourself:

- ✔ How much change do I want to see?
- ✔ How fast do I want these changes to happen?
- ✔ How will these changes affect my life?

You probably want to see a lot of change unfold in a short amount of time and have expectations about how your life will drastically improve after these changes happen. ('When I lose these ten pounds, I will be happier, attract a partner and find a better job!') Although many positive changes most certainly do take place when you achieve your health goals, you don't magically turn into a different person and assume a radically different life. As the saying states: 'Wherever you go, there you are.'

Some questions to ask yourself about your expectations of mindful eating are:

- ✔ Am I clear about what I'm expecting to gain or what I'm hoping to achieve through mindful eating?
- ✔ Where did these expectations come from? What are they based on?
- ✔ Are my expectations clouding my experience of the present moment?
- ✔ Do I feel like this approach is a sustainable solution?

Performing a reality check

If you're hoping that mindful eating offers you quick-fix weight loss, you may be sorely disappointed when I tell you that you're looking in the wrong place. Mindfulness is a slow and steady approach to cultivating a long-term, positive, healthy and balanced relationship with food.

Although mindfulness sounds very simple – and indeed in many ways it truly is – don't be fooled. Part of the challenge lies within its simplicity. Just paying attention is so simple, but how often do you forget to do it? Simple does not necessarily equate to easy; nobody ever said that just because mindfulness is simple that it's going to be an effortless path or journey to embark on. Mindful eating, like any kind of training in mindfulness, requires effort, consistent dedication, commitment and practice. At times it can and will challenge you.

Try to notice, observe and be open to whatever unfolds for you in this journey. When you don't have expectations you can remain open to all surprises and you don't have an attachment to a future outcome. It helps to keep you in the present moment. Look at your mindful eating journey as an experiment, and you're the unbiased scientist or researcher remaining neutral to the results. This thought experiment is a mindfulness practice in itself because it allows you to bear witness to what's unfolding in the present moment without being attached to it. You're less likely to get swept up by your thoughts and emotions, and you can simply be present for whatever you're experiencing.

Patience helps you on this journey towards mindful awareness. Every time you notice yourself having unrealistically high expectations, remind yourself that 'slow and steady wins the race'.

Considering what you can expect

On the other side of the equation, you don't want to set unrealistically low expectations that don't encourage you to make an effort to achieve what you want.

Some realistic expectations that you can set for mindful eating are:

- ✔ I realize that mindful eating isn't about getting it right; it's about being present and aware for whatever is arising. There's no such thing as being good or bad at it.

- ✔ I know that mindful eating may or may not lead to weight loss, but it certainly contributes to a holistic approach to weight loss.

- ✔ Discovering how to eat mindfully is only part of the equation of living a healthy lifestyle. If I have health goals, I also need to take into consideration how to manage my stress levels and emotions, and how much sleep and exercise I am getting.

- ✔ Mindful eating is a long-term practice. It is not a quick-fix solution to healing, balancing and establishing a positive relationship with food.

- ✔ Over time and with practice I will deepen my understanding of all that mindful eating encompasses.

- ✔ I will gradually be able to let go of my unrealistic expectations around mindful eating.

- ✔ There's no such thing as being perfect at mindful eating. Over time I will increase my present-moment awareness around food, but I can still expect to have some mindless eating moments.

- ✔ Sometimes eating mindfully will be emotionally or mentally challenging.

- ✔ Mindful eating may occasionally feel pointless or a waste of my time. At these times I will remind myself of why I want to begin to eat more mindfully.

> ✔ Practicing patience will be extremely helpful to me on this journey.
>
> ✔ Discovering how to be more accepting and kind towards myself will help me cultivate a more positive relationship with food.
>
> ✔ The more I practice mindful eating, the more it will become second nature to me.
>
> ✔ Even when I'm dedicated to mindful eating, my mind will wander; this is human and to be expected.
>
> ✔ Mindful eating requires a daily commitment, but even if I veer from the path, I can at any moment choose to come back to a mindful way of eating and living.
>
> ✔ The benefits and rewards I experience from mindful eating may be hard to see at first.
>
> ✔ I need to be flexible with my approach and adapt any mindful eating techniques to work best for me.

After reading this list, look back at your own expectations and ask yourself how realistic they are. Do they need some adjusting?

Identifying your health goals

Realistic expectations, in the form of goals and objectives, can become a handy roadmap to help you get to where you want to go. This may seem paradoxical and at odds with mindfulness, since the practice of mindfulness is rooted in the present moment and goal setting focuses on the future. However, you can reap the benefits of goal setting, since it's been shown to help people initiate and follow through on change, while at the same time staying present and focused on the here and now with acceptance and non-judgment.

The term *goal setting* is imbued with striving and trying to get to a future point in time at the expense of experiencing the present moment. If you have a tendency to be overly strict or harsh with yourself, then perhaps try setting a health aspiration.

Setting an *aspiration* means that you're setting a heartfelt hope or wish to achieve something – it invites a softer attitude and is more aligned with the mindful eating mindset outlined in Chapter 5. An *aspiration* instead of a *goal* allows you to loosen your grip on the outcome, release the need for hyper-vigilant control and relax into the process.

Sometimes when you try to make changes too fast, you see an unexpected backlash, especially if you're not doing the inner groundwork to accompany the outer changes. Mindfulness helps you determine the speed at which those changes are best made to help you achieve your long-term health goals.

Now that you've fine-tuned your expectations, it's time to set some mindful eating goals (or if you prefer . . . aspirations)!

Start small at first. Like developing all new habits, set realistic aspirations that you know you can achieve.

When it comes to setting goals, remember to make them:

- ✔ **Specific**: Some examples are: sit down when eating; turn off the TV when eating; if you're being distracted by conversation, put down your fork; eat with chopsticks to remind yourself to slow down; put your fork down between bites; pause for one minute before you eat.

- ✔ **Time-oriented**: One mindful meal *per day*, or three *per week* for example.

- ✔ **Obtainable**: Is what you laid out for yourself realistically obtainable? Setting the aspiration to eat one mindful meal per day or several mindful meals a week is reasonable, but setting the aspiration that you'll never eat mindlessly ever again is not.

- ✔ **Positive**: Keep goals focused on the positive rather than the negative. For example, instead of saying, *I'll never eat chocolate chip cookies right out of the bag again* say, *The next time I want cookies, I'll portion them out on a plate and be fully present for the experience.*

- ✔ **Flexible:** Rather than imposing rigid rules, allow flexibility and account for adaptability. For example, instead of saying, *I never* or *I only* shift the vocabulary to *I set the intention to try . . .* or *I will do my best given the situation to. . . .*

In your mindful eating journal write down the top three goals (aspirations) that you hope to achieve through discovering how to eat mindfully.

Replacing mindless with mindful eating habits

Use your mindful eating journal to brainstorm the mindless eating habits that are unsupportive in the lifestyle that you want to create for yourself and that you are ready to let go of and change. List whatever comes to mind. Is it eating really late at night? How about frequent snacking between meals? Is it eating out more than you like or chronically overeating in restaurants? After you brainstorm your list, circle the top three mindless eating habits that you want to change.

Next to each *mindless* eating habit, write your ideal *mindful* eating replacement. Look at the following examples in Table 4-2:

Table 4-2   Mindless versus Mindful Eating Habits

Mindless Eating Habit	Mindful Eating Habit
Eating on the run.	I will do my best to eat sitting down at a table.
Mindless distracted eating in front of the TV or computer.	I will do my best to remove all distractions and focus on my food while I eat.
Eating to avoid feeling an unpleasant emotion.	I will try to become more mindful of how I'm feeling and make an effort to find out how to work with my emotions directly rather than cover over them with food.

More often than not, you start out with good intentions about wanting to establish health changes, yet one of the top reasons people don't follow through on goals is because they simply forget! You forget your goals for all sorts of reasons, such as because you have too many things going on at once, or you're tired or stressed.

How can you trigger yourself to remember to act on your mindful eating replacements? What kind of reminder can you set that helps you remember to eat sitting down or to eat without distractions? Maybe you can set a reminder on your phone (but remember, try not to eat while being distracted by your phone!). Or perhaps write these three new aspirations on a piece of paper and place them in a highly visible place, such as on your bathroom mirror or fridge door.

The good news is that simply thinking about and writing down the mindless eating habits that you want to change and thinking about how you want to replace the mindless tendency with a more mindful one is an excellent place to start.

Planning for failure

Another trick to help steer you in the right direction towards achieving your goals is to plan for failure. You may think: 'Why on earth do I want to think about failure?' Actually, research shows that planning for failure – making a list of all the things that may get in the way of you and your goal and coming up with strategies to prevent those things from happening – helps people achieve their goals more than if they didn't plan for failure.

Think about what triggers you to throw mindful eating out the window and fall back into your old habitual mindless ways. Next to each of your goals, make a note of what is the most likely thing to throw you off course. Here's an example:

Goal	*Triggers for Slip-ups*	*Back-up Prevention Plan*
Eat without distractions for one meal a day.	TV in kitchen is often my primary distraction.	Remove TV from kitchen or throw a towel over it before I eat. Reminder: visual cue; leave towel on kitchen chair or next to TV.

It's the path, not the destination: Focusing on the present

Mindfulness is not about arriving at your destination – believing that over there is better than right here. This belief leads you to live in the future. For example, always thinking about how when you lose that extra weight *then* you can be happy, enjoy life, have fun and love yourself – but not until you get there. The mindful path brings your focus back to the present moment, allowing you to simply enjoy your life as it is now.

Chapter 5

Cultivating a Supportive Mindful Eating Mindset

I'm going to let you in on a secret: your current attitude is more important and more valuable to you than what you did or didn't do in the past, how much you know about mindful eating and what your current circumstances are.

Cultivating a positive mindset is enormously beneficial for your mindful eating journey. The good news is that you can choose what attitude you want to embrace in your life – even on a moment-to-moment basis.

A mindset is an established set of mental attitudes. The different attitudes that you foster and strengthen together make up what is referred to as your mindset. In this chapter I explore the attitudes that support eating mindfully.

Cultivating Your Garden of Mindful Attitudes

Just as your behavior can become automatic and mindless, as I explain in Chapter 3, so too can your attitudes and thought patterns. Awareness is just as essential to changing attitudes as it is to changing habits. (Flip to Chapter 4 for more on awareness as the first key to change.)

Think of your mind as a garden: awareness as the fertile soil and positive attitudes as the seeds you plant to support your mindful eating journey. As you plant and cultivate the seeds of acceptance, non-judgment, letting go, curiosity and openness, compassion and gratitude, you eventually reap the benefits of living in a beautiful garden – hopefully one that bears delicious fruit! These beautiful plants, your new attitudes, create a positive environment for your mindfulness practice to flourish.

All of these attitudes overlap and interconnect with each other. The essence of what is referred to as mindfulness encompasses and embodies all of these attitudes, and they're at the heart of mindfulness practice.

Indulging acceptance

Mindfulness and acceptance go hand in hand. When you're mindful, with full awareness of the present moment, you fully accept what you're experiencing without the labeling, judging, resisting, pushing and pulling that often accompany your experience.

Acceptance is a tricky concept for a lot of people to grasp. They often think of acceptance as 'giving up' or 'resignation'. But acceptance, in this sense, refers not to passively accepting, but actively acknowledging and being present for what is. If the word acceptance is hard to accept, then think of acceptance as simply acknowledging instead, if this word is easier to accept!

Acceptance also doesn't mean approving or condoning what's happening in the present moment. It's not saying, 'This is okay,' or 'I'm okay with the way this is.' Acceptance is about *not arguing* with what is and simply witnessing it with openness, non-judgment and curiosity. With acceptance, you open to things as they are by saying: 'I'm in this situation. I don't approve of it. I don't think it's okay, but it is what it is, and I can't change that it happened, so I may as well move forward from here.'

The practice of mindfulness can help foster acceptance (and vice versa) because as you start to observe the present moment with non-judgment, you begin to embrace it for what it is: this is acceptance.

Acceptance and loving what is

I think of acceptance as *loving what is*, a saying popularized by author and spiritual teacher Byron Katie. Loving what is means you're embracing and accepting the present moment, because if you don't accept it, you're not living in reality but in fantasy or your imagination. Essentially, non-acceptance equates to resistance; it's like trying to swim against the tide when you can more easily conserve your energy by going with the flow.

In her book *Loving What Is: How Four Questions Can Change Your Life* (Harmony House, 2002), Byron Katie says: 'I'm a lover of what is, not because I'm a spiritual person, but because it hurts when I argue with reality. We can know that reality is good just as it is, because when we argue with it, we experience tension and frustration. We don't feel natural or balanced. When we stop opposing reality, action becomes simple, fluid, kind, and fearless.'

Although acceptance doesn't magically make everything better, consider the alternative consequences of non-acceptance: you're engaging in a fight you're guaranteed to lose! You don't have to like what's happening in the present moment, but you're willing to work with it as it is, essentially dropping the fight. This is where approaching the present moment with curiosity, compassion and non-judgment also comes in handy.

Acceptance means dodging the second arrow

The practice of acceptance can be extremely supportive of starting to eat more mindfully. How so? Oftentimes when people feel a sense of discomfort, pain or an unpleasant feeling, they try to distract themselves, or avoid or numb this feeling by using food – and not usually in a mindful manner. Sound familiar? This approach can ultimately cause more suffering – it's like heaping a nice big pile of struggle on top of your already existing suffering. The Buddha called this type of response the second arrow. If you work directly with what you're initially feeling, however painful the feeling is (the first arrow), then you don't have to cause yourself more suffering by turning to ice cream to make yourself feel better or binging on food (the second arrow).

The second arrow can often come in the form of fear-based thoughts. After you mindlessly overeat, for example, you drown yourself in thoughts of guilt, blame and shame. Thoughts arise like, 'I can't believe I did this again. I'm such a terrible person!' These thoughts are all second (third, fourth and fifth) arrows that only perpetuate cycles of suffering. By accepting that you just mindlessly overate, you can prevent or stop that downward spiral and simply notice what you did, recognize that it's now in the past and you can't change it, and move forward from there. In this new moment, you can choose new thoughts and actions that are more supportive of your health and wellbeing.

Accepting what you can change

Are you familiar with the well-known serenity prayer by American theologian Reinhold Niebuhr? It goes like this:

> *God grant me the serenity to accept the things I cannot change, the courage to change the things I can, and wisdom to know the difference.*

That's some timeless wisdom right there. When it comes to acceptance, it's helpful to know the difference between what's in your power to change and what's not. If it's raining outside, you really can't do anything about it, so you may as well accept it! Getting caught up in thoughts of 'Oh I wish it wasn't raining! Why does it have to rain today? This isn't fair!' only causes you more suffering, and what's the point of that? What does that accomplish for you? Instead, you can acknowledge that it's raining and make sure you grab your raincoat and umbrella on the way out! Being aware that you can't control everything and accepting that is a huge help!

Accepting yourself

Acceptance is also really helpful when it comes to working with body image. Many people have quite distorted body images that have potentially damaging long-term consequences. Embracing an attitude of acceptance towards your body helps support you on your mindful eating journey. No matter how much you try, you can't change how tall you are, your shoe size, the color of your eyes, or the shape of your face, to name just a few features. Accept and know the difference between what you can and can't change. Do you think that spending your time wishing that you were different makes matters better or worse for yourself? (Look out for that second arrow again!) It can also prove to be psychologically and emotionally harmful. You may even take this hurt out on yourself by harming your body physically through overeating or underfeeding, or depriving yourself of happiness by staying at home because of your non-acceptance of the way you look.

When it comes to things that you do have an influence over, like your weight, for example, acceptance still comes in handy. If you're 25 pounds overweight, wishing that you weren't isn't going to help you. Arguing with your body or thinking mean thoughts about your body is surely only going to make matters worse. However, acknowledging that you're overweight and no longer want to feel the consequences of that empowers you to move in the direction you want to move in. Not accepting it keeps you stuck in the same place, while accepting it allows you to mindfully move forward.

If you spend all your time and energy fighting against what is, then you're not going to have any energy to actually take the steps to change it!

Although it feels counterintuitive, establishing the changes you long to make becomes easier when you embrace an attitude of acceptance. That's why so many programs for change, including the well-known Alcoholics Anonymous 12-step program, incorporate acceptance. As many people acknowledge, the first step is admitting you have a problem. This is acceptance.

Grab your mindful eating journal and write down what it is that you find difficult to accept about yourself or your body. (Check out Chapter 4 on how to start a mindful eating journal.) Is holding on to this thought causing you more suffering or is it helping you and making your life more enjoyable? Can you see a reason to hold on to this thought? Do you really know that this thought is objectively true and not just your own perception?

Come up with an affirmation that feels realistic and believable. Write the affirmation on a card and place the card in a visible location as a reminder to stay in an attitude of acceptance. Maybe the affirmation, 'I accept myself completely' is difficult for you to believe at this point in time, so you can write something like 'I accept myself in this moment' if you prefer.

Acceptance encompasses self-love, compassion and kindness. Accepting yourself unconditionally is what the Tibetan Buddhist tradition calls *maitri,* translated as *loving-kindness* or *unconditional friendliness.*

Embracing non-judgment

The attitude of non-judgment goes hand in hand with acceptance. Non-judgment is about being a neutral observer. Sometimes (oftentimes . . . perhaps almost all the time) you get lost in your judgments, constantly labeling everything as good or bad, right or wrong. As with acceptance, you need to simply acknowledge that the present moment is what it is and things are what they are without putting an added layer of judgments on top of it.

Judging the different judgments

If you look up the word *judgment* generally two meanings are given. The first one refers to judging a situation. Your mind is naturally judgmental. You evolved this capacity as an essential survival mechanism. In primitive times, if you approached a tribe of people you hadn't seen before, your brain assessed the situation for danger. You thought, 'Are they friendly or are they going to kill me?'

Even today you're constantly scanning and judging your environment, including the people in it, for information about your own survival and safety – even if it's regarding the safety of protecting your social status or image! Your brain is geared towards finding fault with situations so it can try to problem solve and pre-empt dangers before they happen. So you're already geared towards a critical judgmental mind, which brings us to the second definition – being overly critical or judgmental of people, places, situations and oftentimes yourself, in an unhelpful way.

Use curiosity as a powerful antidote to prevent or shift constant judgment. Check out the section 'Cultivating curiosity and openness' later in this chapter to find out more about developing curiosity.

You can judge a situation and make discerning choices without being critical of it. Judging to assess a situation is one thing, but chronically judging life in a critical manner creates unnecessary suffering. This kind of judging often implies that you're not satisfied with the situation and you'd rather it be different than the way it is. This brings us back to non-acceptance and arguing with what is.

Non-judgment towards ourselves

Beware of being judgmental about yourself and your own behavior. Judgment is not a reflection on others; it's a reflection of you and your own mind, beliefs and perceptions. Practicing non-judgment goes hand in hand with acceptance. Becoming more accepting of yourself and not harboring self-judgment is how you learn to be more self-compassionate.

The practice of non-judgment allows you to experience your moment-to-moment reality with openness and acceptance. Practicing non-judgment allows you to have an open mind rather than a narrow mind when approaching life. You stay open to different ideas, thoughts, concepts and people.

Being a mindful observer of your own thoughts is a great place to start. The next time you notice yourself harboring self-judgment, simply take your thought and imagine transporting it to a cloud passing by in the sky. You have no attachment to that cloud; it's simply a thought-cloud passing by that you can bear witness to.

The next time you notice yourself judging an aspect of your relationship with food and mentally labeling it, ask yourself: 'Is this really true?' If you catch yourself judging a food as 'good' or 'bad', ask yourself where this belief comes from and see if you can loosen the grip of judgment and have a more direct experience with food, eating and your body without the need to add additional layers.

It's an Unfortunate Fortune

There was once a very poor family living on a small farm in ancient China. One day a beautiful wild horse, worth a sizable fortune, came galloping onto the land. The farmer's son was excited and exclaimed joyfully, yet to his surprise, the father looked at him and said: 'Who knows if this is good or bad? We shall see.'

The next day the horse ran off, and the boy lamented that the family had fallen back into misfortune. 'Who knows?' the father said, 'we shall see.' On the third day the horse returned with a herd of six other horses. The young boy jumped up and down shouting, 'We're rich! We're rich! Lucky us!' The young boy decided to ride one of the horses before the family was due to sell it on the fourth day. The boy fell off the horse and broke his leg very badly. As the rest of the family wept for

their misfortune, the father remained unwavering as he said, 'Who knows if this is good or bad? We shall see.' The next day war broke out in the country and many troops came to their village to recruit new soldiers – but the boy was spared because of his broken leg.

The purpose of this ancient Buddhist parable is to show that you can never truly know what is good or bad; a situation's only as good or bad as you perceive it to be. When you label something as bad can you absolutely know that this is true? You hold on to your attachments of what you want or don't want to happen, but you can never fully understand how things will turn out in the end. By embracing an attitude of non-judgment, you can spare yourself unnecessary suffering.

We can't ever know if something is really good or bad, it's only our perceptions that make it so. (Check out the nearby sidebar, 'It's an Unfortunate Fortune' for more on this idea.)

Discovering how to let go

Whatever baggage you've been lugging around with you, day after day – and I don't just mean physical – it's time to let it go! Wanting to hold onto things is a natural tendency. You constantly tell yourself stories in your mind about things that happened, how they shouldn't have happened, how you wish something else had happened . . . you get the picture.

When you become fixated on a story-line in your mind, you miss the present moment. When you're not accepting the present moment, you're wishing it were different. Letting go allows you to release the non-acceptance and embrace what is with open arms.

Letting go and impermanence

Letting go can be viewed as the essence of mindfulness. You observe each moment as it arises and then let it go to make way for the new moment showing up. Letting go relates to the concept of impermanence, a core idea in Buddhist teachings. Even though you know that everything is constantly changing, impermanence is quite hard to grasp emotionally because you're hardwired for security. Constant change means that you can't hold on forever to your loved ones, your job, your home, special moments and even your own life! Realizing that all these special things will eventually pass is challenging and even painful.

Every moment is fleeting, which is why you want to be present for all that each moment offers. Traditional wisdoms like Buddhism teach that everything eventually passes, and, instead of embracing this truth, most people struggle against it, clinging to things and attachments and holding on rather than letting go.

Letting go and your relationship with food

Take a moment to think about how you can practice letting go when it comes to your relationship with food. Although everyone can learn to let go, this practice is especially important for people who are overly rigid, controlling, hyper-vigilant or restrictive about food and eating.

Identify the controller within you. Take a moment to pause and reflect on the following yes or no questions. Does this sound like you?

- ✔ I constantly count nutrients (calories, grams of fat, carbohydrates, and so on) to make sure that I stay within the safe zone with my diet.

- ✔ I weigh myself at least every day to make sure that I don't go over my desired limit.

✔ I can't trust myself to eat bad foods because I'm scared that I'll spiral out of control.

✔ If I have a bad eating day, I tend to overeat at night.

✔ I need to make sure that I have a perfect day of eating.

✔ I don't like other people preparing my food. I need to do it myself.

✔ I feel that it's unacceptable if I overeat.

If you answered yes to any of these questions, consider exploring the practice of letting go.

When it comes to your relationship with food, you can start to let go of many different things. Some of these include:

✔ **Letting go of the need to control:** situations involving food, people and outcomes.

✔ **Letting go of the need for more:** always thinking about wanting more food, even before you've finished what you're currently eating.

✔ **Letting go of attachments:** to specific desires and wants, and outcomes.

✔ **Letting go of the past:** the stories that continue to circle around and around in your mind that are no longer serving you.

✔ **Letting go of outdated ideas, beliefs and thought patterns:** concepts that were passed down to you or that you perhaps picked up as a young child that no longer serve you.

✔ **Letting go of destructive emotions:** these include letting go of the perpetuation of guilt, shame, blame, criticism, anger and even fear.

✔ **Letting go of striving:** letting go of living in the future, to get to a better now.

✔ **Letting go of addictions and behavioral patterns:** including any habits that are no longer serving you and the life you want to live.

Letting go doesn't mean that you can't set goals and intentions, make affirmations and then take action. It does, however, require letting go of the outcome and trusting that it's all going to be okay. Letting go allows you to find that balance between letting things happen and making things happen. Mindfulness can help you recognize where you're trying to exert too much control and help you loosen your grip and relax into the present moment.

Letting go is not condoning or approving of something that happened in the past, but recognizing, with acceptance, that it's now in the past.

Try this short guided visualization on letting go. Start by writing something down that's bothering you or that you're struggling with. It can be anything, big or small. Perhaps someone said something to you that upset you, and you keep replaying it in your mind. Maybe you're holding on to guilt and shame for falling off the wagon and eating something that wasn't within your definition of healthy. Maybe you've been carrying a story around with you since childhood that says you'll never be good enough because your older brother said it on a whim once. It can be anything that you know is no longer serving you and is only causing you unnecessary suffering.

After you've written it down, sit or lie comfortably and close your eyes. Imagine yourself sitting outside on the grass on a beautiful sunny day. You feel calm, peaceful and at ease. You're holding a balloon in your hand. In your mind's eye, you look up. The balloon is carrying the memory of the very thing you're now choosing to let go. With strength, courage and inner guidance, you open your hand to release the balloon. You watch it slowly float up and away from you. The further away it floats from you, the lighter your body feels, freed from that unnecessary memory you're no longer choosing to carry around with you. Rest here for as long as you like, moving slowly and mindfully when you decide to get up again.

When you've finished, take out your mindful eating journal and write down what you experienced during this guided visualization.

Cultivating curiosity and openness

For some reason, as you grow up you tend to become less curious about life.

The beginner's mind

With curiosity, you cultivate a willingness to explore things as they constantly change. You allow yourself to have a beginner's mind. The beginner's mind is like that of a small child, looking at the world with wonder, awe and amazement. But the world didn't become any less amazing as you grew up; your perceptions of reality have changed. When you approach life with a beginner's mind, you also let go of expectations and preconceptions, because you know that every moment is a new moment, completely different than the last.

Curiosity and openness towards your relationship with food

Adopting an attitude of curiosity and openness allows you to uncover insights into your relationship with food and eating. It allows you to ask self-inquiring questions and explore what may have been hidden under the surface for a long time (oftentimes what you stuff down and bury with food).

When you practice curiosity without judgment, you allow yourself the space to be open to the present moment and discover your unfolding relationship with life, which includes your relationship with food.

You can apply curiosity to mindful eating by asking yourself the following questions and noticing what comes up for you.

  ✔ Does this food make me feel more or less tired after I eat it?

  ✔ Is it really in my best long-term interest to continue eating this food?

  ✔ What emotions and thoughts are here with this craving?

  ✔ Do I eat more or less mindlessly when I'm with other people?

  ✔ Why do I tend to eat when I'm stressed out?

You can ask yourself many questions about your relationship with food, eating and your body. Dive in! Get curious and put on your detective's hat. Think of mindful eating as an interesting experiment and observe your behaviors and eating patterns from a non-judgmental point-of-view that allows space for change to emerge. From this stance you can see what works and what doesn't. Curiosity cultivates awareness, and awareness is the first key to change. (Chapter 4 has more on the four keys to change.)

Curiosity also helps you to keep mindfully aware of your senses. In fact, when you cultivate curiosity in the moment, you're automatically and intuitively practicing mindfulness! You can engage your curiosity and openness by exploring:

✔ What does this food really taste like?

✔ What does it smell like?

✔ What does this food have to offer visually?

Showing up in the present moment means that you're willing to explore your life with a sense of openness that naturally ties into acceptance and non-judgment.

Developing Self-compassion

Do you think you need a little motivation to help you on your mindful eating journey? Well, guess what? Motivation is readily at your disposal, and the good news is that you don't need to play the drill sergeant or inner critic to muster it up to help you get started, stay on track or get back on track if you veer from the path.

Why self-compassion trumps self-criticism

You may have the mistaken belief that you need to be critical and get tough on yourself when you've done something you feel is not aligned with your goals – especially when it comes to your health. But recent research points counter to this logic: self-compassion as opposed to self-criticism is a far superior strategy to foster motivation – and that's not all. As it turns out, self-compassion also:

✔ Supports the courage and inner strength to follow through on goals and make changes you may have found difficult to make in the past.

✔ Bodes well for fostering self-control and keeping sight of goals.

In fact, the more critical and judgmental you are about yourself, the less likely you are to feel motivated and succeed. Now that's enough of a reason to consciously practice self-compassion!

Want a few more reasons? People who rank high in self-compassion also happen to show many other positive benefits, including:

- ✔ Lower levels of depression
- ✔ Less anxiety
- ✔ Stronger social connections (as opposed to isolation)
- ✔ Less likely to experience eating disorders
- ✔ Tend to be happier and more optimistic overall

On the flip side, self-criticism happens to be negatively associated with these positive, life-enhancing benefits.

Why does self-criticism consistently not work? Because it makes you feel bad! And who wants to feel bad? No one – that's why you turn to things that make you feel better, which often means turning to more food. See how this can create an unpleasant cycle? The antidote is to connect with feeling good by being kind, compassionate and loving with yourself – learning to be your own best supportive friend.

How self-compassion can save you from yourself

Compassion is an awareness of the suffering of others coupled with the desire to relieve it; likewise, just as you wish to relieve the pain of others, self-compassion allows you to be patient, loving, and supportive with yourself.

Self-compassion incorporates mindfulness, self-acceptance, non-judgment and self-kindness. It also encompasses knowing that you're not alone and that other people also experience the challenges and struggles that you do. This is what compassion researcher Kristin Neff calls connecting to our 'shared humanity'. All these components of self-compassion are what prevent it from becoming a ticket for self-indulgence. You may have the mistaken belief that being kind to yourself

Skittles and self-compassion

Still feeling skeptical about whether self-compassion is actually the way to go? A study conducted in 2007 by researchers Claire Adams and Mark Leary from Wake Forest University found that even a minor self-compassion intervention can influence eating habits. The study involved 84 college women who had previously completed a written test to measure their levels of restrictive eating (desire and effort to avoid eating unhealthy foods) and guilty eating (a tendency to feel guilty after eating unhealthily).

The women thought they were taking part in a taste-test experiment and were asked to not eat for two hours before the study. At the beginning of the experiment participants were instructed to drink a full glass of water to clean their palates, when in fact it was to induce a feeling of fullness. Some participants were then asked to eat a doughnut (a food highly recognized as unhealthy and meant to trigger guilt amongst guilty eaters) while they watched an educational video. Members of a control group weren't offered doughnuts.

What happened next is interesting. With members of one group of doughnut-eaters, a researcher came into the room and casually said: '[. . .] several people have told me that they feel bad about eating doughnuts in this study, so I hope you won't be hard on yourself. Everyone eats unhealthily sometimes, and everyone in this study eats this stuff, so I don't think there's any reason to feel really bad about it. This little amount of food doesn't really matter anyway.' However, members of a second group of doughnut-eaters, and the control group, received no such compassionate intervention.

All the participants were then instructed to taste test from three big bowls of candies. They were given a rating sheet and told that they should eat at least one piece of each type of candy, but they could help themselves to as much candy as they wanted.

The researchers found that participants who ranked highly as restrictive and guilty eaters actually ate less with the self-compassion intervention and behaved much like classic non-dieters, reducing food intake after eating the doughnut. Participants who didn't receive the self-compassionate message ate more.

rather than reprimanding yourself is too lenient and is like giving yourself the green light to go out and eat whatever you want. But self-compassion doesn't actually equate to self-indulgence.

In the same way that you would have compassion rather than reprimand a friend who consistently turns to alcohol, you can apply this same level of loving-kindness towards your own eating habits to help steer yourself in the right direction. Self-compassion is about loving yourself so much that you don't want to inflict any kind of suffering on yourself.

One way you can start practicing self-compassion is by becoming aware of your inner critic – the voice within each of us that consistently criticizes everything we do.

To help increase your awareness of the inner critic, for one day, put a coin in a jar every time you have a self-critical thought. To heighten your awareness, count the number of coins at the end of the day. If you have a lot of coins in the jar, don't feel bad about it; most people are surprised at how many times throughout the day they criticize or think negatively of themselves.

Another approach is to make a list in your mindful eating journal of your most chronic self-critical thoughts, such as 'I'm bad', 'I'm stupid' or 'I'm fat'. Now imagine that it was your best friend saying this. Next to each self-critical thought, write down what you would say to your best friend to counteract each of those statements, such as 'You're beautiful exactly the way you are.' Over the next week, choose one of your chronic self-critical thoughts and whenever it comes up, replace it immediately with its positive counterpart. Do the same with your other critical thoughts, and over time their number and frequency will decrease.

The next time you're feeling overly critical or down on yourself for something you just did, try the compassion practice of connecting to the wider shared humanity. Say, for example, that you just over-ate or binged. Take a moment to sit quietly alone and in your mind and heart connect to other people who also feel the same suffering you feel from your struggle with food and send them a wish that they be relieved of it. Send them an aspiration that feels good for you:

> *May you be free from this struggle, may you be happy, may you be healthy, may you find peace.*

Imagine sending them warmth, love and light. Hold this feeling for as long as feels comfortable for you. Then, when you are ready, shift this compassionate feeling towards yourself, repeating the aspiration:

> *May I be free from this struggle, may I be happy, may I be healthy, may I find peace.*

Use whatever aspiration feels good and comes naturally to you. Go at your own pace and explore what comes up for you during this self-compassion and shared humanity exercise.

Fostering an Attitude of Gratitude

Expressing gratitude may just be the simplest way to feel better in any given moment. What a powerful tool! And guess what? It's free and readily at your disposal!

Acknowledging with gratitude all the good in your life is a powerful mindfulness practice that can have far reaching and surprisingly wonderful benefits – especially when it comes to your health. In the realm of psychology, gratitude is consistently associated with greater happiness (just to point out the obvious!). It's also effective at helping foster positive emotions, work through challenging situations, and it can help improve relationships.

Gratitude can help you gain perspective in any situation by:

- ✔ Reminding you of what's really important.
- ✔ Reminding you to focus on the positive.
- ✔ Helping you accept and learn from challenging situations.

If you spend a lot of your time thinking about how much you weigh or how much you don't like something about your body, applying gratitude can help remind you that you can focus on more important things, such as how much you love your family.

When you embrace this attitude, it allows you to look at even the most challenging of situations with gratitude. Some say that you learn your greatest lessons when going through your most difficult times. Even if you struggle with food, your weight or your body, these experiences give you the opportunity to develop and grow. For example, going through the experience of inner strife can teach you about inner peace. Or the experience of feeding yourself poorly (and feeling the consequences of that) can lead to feeding yourself healthfully.

If you struggle with your relationship with food, eating, your weight or your body, think about what you've discovered through these experiences. In your mindful eating journal, write down what these challenges have taught you.

I know many people say that losing weight and keeping it off has been their life-long challenge. If this has been the case for you and you're willing to look at and explore what you've learned through this challenge, some powerful nuggets of wisdom and truth may emerge – and these lessons are definitely something to be grateful for!

The next time you're feeling judgmental towards your body, try to shift gears and apply an attitude of gratitude. Does it feel true for you to express any of these affirmations instead?

- ✔ I'm grateful for all the things my body supports me to do.
- ✔ I'm grateful for what my hands allow me to create.
- ✔ I'm grateful for all the places my feet have carried me to.
- ✔ I'm grateful for all the wonderful smells I've been able to enjoy with my nose.

When it comes to approaching the way you eat, you can easily see the connection between gratitude and food. Food sustains your life. It's what allows you to wake up each and every morning to another miraculous day, another day you have the gift of being alive. Eating offers you sensory pleasure, nourishes and even nurtures you. What a gift to be grateful for!

You may often fall into the trap of considering food as your enemy and express a love-hate relationship with your food. Applying gratitude can help propel a radical shift in your perspective where you just may find a completely new dynamic with your food. Cultivating a balanced, positive and healthy relationship with food is the essence of what mindful eating is all about.

Gratitude is one of the greatest, most profound keys to ending your struggle with food and viewing it as the miracle that it is, helping you to sustain your life.

Chapter 6

Choosing Healthy Foods Mindfully

● ●

In This Chapter

▶ Making smart food choices mindfully

▶ Understanding the difference between real and processed foods

▶ Exploring mindful grocery shopping tips

● ●

*M*indful eating is a non-dietary-specific approach to eating. When it comes to exploring mindful eating, it's not for me to say, 'You should eat this,' or 'You should eat that.' Mindful eating focuses on how and why you eat, rather than on what you eat. What you choose to eat is ultimately up to you, but mindful eating helps you navigate your food choices so that you feel good about the foods you eat. Through the process of mindful eating you start to notice things like, 'This doesn't make me feel good when I eat it,' or 'I feel better when I eat more fruit and less junk food.'

You naturally want to eat better and make smarter food choices because you want to *feel* good. Mindful eating incorporates awareness around informed food choices. In fact, you probably don't realize that some of your food choices are actually promoting mindless rather than mindful eating. In this chapter, I explore some of the basic foundations of making mindfully healthy food choices.

When you begin to eat more mindfully you start to notice body sensations and observe thoughts and emotions before, during, or after you eat, which offer you an opportunity to take a deeper look at your relationship with food. You become aware of how your food choices *affect* you – how food affects the way you feel physically, mentally, emotionally and even, for some people, spiritually.

Taking it one step further and expanding your awareness even more, in this chapter I also consider mindful eating as a reflection of how aware you are of the way your food choices affect the environment.

One Size Doesn't Fit All: Different Approaches to Healthy Eating

Although certain generalizations can be made when it comes to eating (almost everyone can benefit from eating more fruit and vegetables), not one single dietary approach works for everyone. You can actually be healthy within a range of different ways of eating. This is because:

✔ People live in different climates.

✔ People have access to different locally grown foods.

✔ People grow up in different cultures where different foods are preferred over others.

✔ People all have different family experiences and upbringings around food.

✔ People have different food-related belief systems and ethical concerns.

✔ People have different food sensitivities.

✔ People have different preferences, likes and dislikes towards foods.

Although one diet that everyone can follow to the letter may not exist, some things are known for sure, the first one being: the Standard American Diet (SAD), a diet filled with processed foods, heavily based on animal products, refined sugar and excess calories, is not healthy and is actually making a lot of people quite sick.

Blue Zones

We live in a culture obsessed with finding a magic pill for weight loss, youth and longevity. People want to know what the longest-lived people in the world eat. As it turns out, the longest-lived peoples don't share a single diet. They live in various places all over the world in what *New York Times* bestselling author Dan Buettner calls *Blue Zones.* This result shows that you can't boil your health down to 'yogurt or no yogurt', 'fish or no fish', but rather you need to look at the bigger picture that even extends far beyond simply what you choose to eat.

Although many dietary discrepancies exist across the Blue Zones, one common theme was a plant-based diet where minimal calories come from animal products. Some other factors that contributed to Blue Zone longevity include:

✔ Practicing effective stress management.

✔ Incorporating natural movement like walking, hiking and working the land in their lifestyles and living in connection with nature.

✔ Living with a strong sense of purpose.

✔ Living with a sense of faith in the greater mystery of life.

✔ Placing a strong emphasis on the importance of family.

✔ Living within a strong social network.

For more information about Blue Zones, visit Dan Buettner's website www.bluezones.com.

Mindful eating and all the practices and self-reflections outlined in this book help you to tune into your inner body wisdom and choose foods that are the best for you and your body.

Voting with Your Food Dollars

The next time you open your wallet or swipe your card to pay for food, think of each dollar spent as casting a vote, because as you know, money talks. This vote holds a lot of weight because your choice of foods has huge consequences – not just for you and me, but for future generations to come. Every time you buy a food, you're voting for the system that created it and all that goes along with it, including whether it's environmentally supportive or destructive. You're saying, 'Yes, I approve of how this food is produced, I want more of it and I want *you* to supply it to me.'

As a consumer, you get to decide if you want to see more conventional or genetically modified (GM) foods grown or if you want to see more organic farms flourish. You can opt to vote for local, sustainable growing systems that support biodiversity and align in a harmonious way with nature – the choice is yours to make.

The enormity of the consequences of your food choices is alone enough of a reason to eat more mindfully. Considering what's at stake (no pun intended), think carefully about just how your food choices impact the world around you.

Navigating the current food environment is very confusing, with so many food products stocking the shelves. In the opening line of his book *In Defense of Food* (Penguin Books, 2009) famous food journalist Michael Pollan advised 'Eat food. Not too much. Mostly plants,' which is an excellent guide to choosing what to eat.

In the rest of this chapter, I explore what these choices look like and why you need a food journalist to point out the definition of *food* – and by that I mean *real* food (as opposed to the processed food products you've become accustomed to identifying as 'food'). The good news is that the healthiest foods are also the ones with the lowest environmental impact and ecological footprint.

The other healthy food guidelines that I explore in this chapter include: whole (real) food, sustainable, local, organic and plant foods. When you choose to buy these foods, you're casting a vote for:

- ✔ Your health (not only physical health, but the mental, emotional and even the spiritual health of you and your family).
- ✔ Your local community.
- ✔ The environment.

Exploring these healthy food criteria and making conscious food choices can be part of exploring *why* you eat. For example, you may choose to eat a vegan or vegetarian diet because you don't want to support the factory farming of animals – a powerful *why* indeed!

Vote for real food

Once upon a time there was no need to distinguish between real food and imitation food, or what Michael Pollan calls *food-like substances*. Many of the 'foods' included in the 43,000 products that the average grocery store carries more closely resemble man-made products than foods found in nature. If you walked around the grocery store with your great-grandmother (or grandmother) she wouldn't recognize half the items in there. Most food offered for sale today is undoubtedly a far cry from what our ancestors used to eat.

The power of processed

Processed foods made by large food companies are designed with one thing in mind – profits. And in order to reap maximum profits, companies manipulate their products to have a long shelf life. The result of refinement is food that is stripped of certain nutrients yet full of added weird chemicals, preservatives and food additives to reach the desired state. Foods are also engineered to have a more desirable mouth-feel to make the eating experience more pleasurable, increasing the chance that you buy the product again.

Food companies have spent billions (with a *B*) of dollars on finding the perfect bliss point – the right combination of the Big Three (sugar, fat and salt) that triggers the pleasure center of the brain. When your brain's pleasure center is hyper-stimulated (as it is when you eat foods high in sugar, fat and salt), it is very difficult for you to stop eating, even after you're stuffed full. Some of these food products now more closely resemble a drug than real food and are prompting a huge new wave of what some researchers are calling food addiction.

Processed foods are often made with:

- ✔ Low-quality, cheap ingredients
- ✔ Refined ingredients
- ✔ Non-organic (and possibly genetically modified) ingredients

✔ Untested preservatives and additives

✔ Synthetic, man-made ingredients

✔ Chemicals and food dyes

The next time you're trying to decide if something is a real food or not, ask yourself if this food is found in nature as is, or if it had to go through a major (often industrial) process first.

A perfect example that illustrates the difference between processed foods versus homemade whole-food alternatives is shown in Table 6-1 below. The first column shows a store-bought guacamole, the second is a list of ingredients to make your own homemade guacamole. Check out the incredibly long list of ingredients in the first column – over 45 of them! For guacamole? Do you recognize these ingredients? Now look at the homemade version. What differences do you notice between the two?

Table 6-1	Store-bought Guacamole versus Homemade Guacamole
Processed Version	**Homemade with whole foods**
Skim milk, Soybean oil, Tomatoes, Water, Hydrogenated vegetable oil (Coconut oil, safflower and/or corn oil), Contains less than 2% avocado, Eggs, Onion*, Salt, Distilled vinegar, Egg yolks, Sugar, Nonfat dry milk, Whey (milk), Lactic acid, Sodium casein-ate (milk), Soy protein isolate, Tomato juice, Mono and diglycerides, Spices, Sodium benzoate, Potassium sorbate, Gelatin, Corn starch, Guar gum, Cellulose gel, Cellulose gum, Mustard flour, Black pepper, Oregano, Thyme, Bay leaf, Red chili pepper, Lemon juice concentrate, Locust bean gum, Disodium phosphate, Gum Arabic, Xanthan gum, Cilantro*, Calcium chloride, Natural Flavors, Extractive of garlic, black pepper and paprika oil, Citric acid, Ascorbic acid, Dextrose, Artificial colors (Blue 1, Red 40, Yellow 5, Yellow 6), *Dehydrated. Contains: MILK, EGG SOYBEAN	Avocado, Freshly squeezed lemon juice, Diced tomatoes, Garlic and onion (optional), Fresh cilantro (coriander)

You may need a little practice or reorganization to get into the swing of preparing your own foods at home, but really, it's simpler than you may think. Just look at the homemade version of guacamole above – that's a five-minute recipe right there!

Choosing nutritious food

There is hope. Real food still exists. It makes up a small percentage of what you find in the grocery store, but with a little guidance, you'll be well equipped to choose what is rightfully yours, and what nature has to offer you – the gift of real food.

Whole food

Whole food is just that – whole. According to the dictionary it is: *food that has been processed or refined as little as possible and is free from additives or other artificial substances.* It's a one-ingredient food, no ingredients list required: cherries, peaches, apples, pumpkin, bananas, tomatoes, and the list goes on. With whole-food ingredients, you can prepare whole-food meals. See Chapter 7 for more on mindful meal preparation.

Although whole foods don't come with an ingredients list, in some countries, like Canada and the US, if you look closely, they come with a little sticker with numbers on it called a PLU sticker, which you need to read! (Check with your government health authorities for deciphering code labels on produce in your country and double check on labeling laws for organic produce.) This code lets you know whether this food is conventionally grown, organic or genetically modified (gasp!). Check out the chart later in this chapter to find out how to decode the codes.

A further word of caution: some countries don't have strict labeling laws around the use of the term 'whole food' on package labels. Use common sense and read ingredients. Don't take nutritional claims on the front of packages at face value.

Nutrient-dense foods

Nutrient-dense foods are foods that have a high ratio of nutrients to calories. Foods that have few nutrients to calories are known as energy-dense foods. Empty calorie foods are foods that are highly processed, have few nutrients and lots of calories.

Noodling around

When it comes to eating more whole foods, sometimes it's just a matter of a little creativity and thinking outside of the conventional box. Have you ever tried to make a one-ingredient noodle? It's easy, no cooking required; after all, it's only one ingredient! For this noodle idea, you'll have to buy (or borrow) a spiral slicer, a handy kitchen tool I highly recommend. All you have to do is place a zucchini (courgette) – washed and preferably organic – into the spiral slicer and away you go – turning the handle to create instant noodles!

Thank goodness that the most nutrient-dense foods around happen to be the most tasty and delicious. Can you guess which foods are the more nutrient dense? Fruit and vegetables! On the other hand, processed foods tend to be more energy dense – not good for your health, or your waistline.

Taking a step in the right direction

Take a step in the right direction and move closer towards real, whole foods at a pace that you feel comfortable with. You'll find a wide range in the quality of ingredients in food products. If you normally buy regular white pasta, try buying a quinoa pasta instead, or even better, try making your own zucchini (courgette) pasta as a whole-food alternative to store-bought noodles. (Check out the nearby sidebar 'Noodling around'.)

Vote for plants

Nutrition debates abound; yet none are more intense and emotionally charged than the meat-eating versus vegetarian debate, with arguments supporting both sides of the equation. Ultimately deciding what to eat is up to you, but taking the following factors into consideration is worthwhile:

- ✔ Much research points to the benefits of eating plant-based diets and reducing animal-based protein intake. However, some research shows that small amounts of animal products (especially fish) may be okay to include and has led to a new way of eating called *flexitarian*, a predominantly vegetarian diet with the occasional addition of small amounts of animal products.

✔ If you eat a heavy meat-based diet, buying from local, organic sources is important. Go for quality over quantity. If you're buying store-bought conventional meat, then remember that you're voting for the many factory farms that contribute to environmental devastation, including the pollution and contamination of the local water supply, the use of pharmaceuticals, antibiotics and growth hormones (which also enter the water supply), as well as the inhumane living conditions of millions of animals.

✔ Fruit and vegetables offer the best, most complete sources of minerals, vitamins, fiber, phytonutrients, enzymes and co-enzymes, are low in calories and saturated fats and actually provide a lot more protein than most people think.

✔ A plant-based diet is more environmentally friendly than a diet heavy in animal products. According to statistics, for every pound of beef you choose not to eat, you save anywhere from 2,500 to 5,000 gallons of water, and eating one pound of hamburger does the same damage to the environment as driving your car for more than three weeks!

When it comes down to it, fruits, vegetables and plant foods are an excellent choice, not only for your health, but also for the health of the environment as well.

If you're a meat eater and would like to slowly transition to a vegan or vegetarian diet, you can take small steps in the directions you wish to go in, one day at a time.

Vote for sustainability

Mindful eating embodies your relationship with where the food that you eat comes from and how it was produced. When was the last time you looked at your dinner and wondered how far it had to come or how destructive the impact of your food choice was on the environment? This contemplation is an essential component to mindful eating.

The definition of sustainable food includes:

✔ Producing food that is healthy for both humans and animals.

✔ Practicing food growing methods that don't harm the environment, but rather enhance it or harmonize with it.

✔ Using non-renewable resources in the most efficient way.

✔ Providing humane working conditions and fair wages for farm workers and a fair return for the farmers.

✔ Respecting animals.

✔ Helping local communities by supporting local farmers and keeping your money in the community.

The essence of sustainable farming is how you choose to treat the environment, working with, not against, the laws of nature and natural resources. This kind of farming keeps the environment healthy and uses natural solutions that enable economically viable food production.

Many conventional farming practices deplete rather than enhance natural resources through soil degradation, chemical pollution, pollution of groundwater, loss of biodiversity and the enormous use of fossil-fuel energy.

One of the changes you can make immediately to help support the environment is to choose local and organic foods.

Vote for local

Luckily, new groups of people are sprouting up, redefining the way that they eat to make a statement about the increasing disconnect between the mass population and their food sources. New terms are being used such as *locavore* (a person whose diet consists primarily of locally grown foods) and *the 100-mile diet* (a diet using only foods produced from within a 100-mile radius).

If you've had the pleasure of experiencing a freshly picked salad, then you know what I'm talking about when I say it's simply incomparable to most store-bought produce. The juiciness, the vibrancy of the colors, the freshness, the tenderness of the greens – now that's worth being present for!

Local foods:

- ✔ **Reduce your ecological footprint:** Food travels on average about 1,300 miles from farm to table.

- ✔ **Are fresh:** Locally grown foods are usually sold within one day of being harvested. The quality and freshness of the ingredients you work with in the kitchen is drastically improved, and the ingredients also have a higher nutrient content than their older counterparts.

- ✔ **Have more variety:** Most varieties of fresh produce sold in stores have been bred for their commercial properties, often at the expense of their taste. Most people don't realize that there are dozens, even hundreds, of varieties of common crops such as tomatoes and cucumbers. Local farmers often grow varieties for the quality of their taste, and you can try heirloom varieties you've probably never even heard of!

- ✔ **Are convenient:** With more and more local farm shops and farmers' markets popping up all over the world, especially in North America, it's becoming increasingly easy to buy locally and sustainably grown organic foods. Food co-ops and CSAs are also a great way to have convenient access to local foods. (See the later section 'Exploring your alternatives to the supermarket' for more on these.)

- ✔ **Connect you with the farmer:** You can develop a wonderful connection with the farmers providing you and your family with healthy, wholesome food.

- ✔ **Reduce waste:** Less packaging means less garbage, and less garbage helps ease the overflowing burden on landfills and the excessive waste issue. More whole foods mean more compost waste and more enriched soil!

Vote for organic

Organic food – what once seemed like a hippie trend in the seventies and eighties has now become a mainstay in our culture. More recent awareness around the devastating effects of conventional farming practices have led to an explosion in demand for organically grown food; it is the fastest growing segment in the American food industry, growing by about 20 percent per year. How's that for voting with your food dollars!

Some of the many benefits of buying organic food include eating food that:

✔ Contains no pesticides, synthetic and chemical fertilizers.

✔ Is better for the environment (grown with natural fertilizers, weeds and insects are controlled naturally).

✔ Is safely produced, as organically raised animals are not given antibiotics, growth hormones or fed animal byproducts.

Avoiding the Dirty Dozen

When it comes to buying non-organic, some foods are worse than others. The Environmental Working Group (EWG) has compiled a list of the dirtiest conventionally grown foods, the Dirty Dozen (although they list 15 foods – I guess they just liked the sound of it!). These foods are often the most heavily sprayed with herbicides and pesticides. For the love of food, your body and the planet, do your mighty best to buy these foods organic! The EWG also list what they call the Clean Fifteen (of which there are actually 15 foods), which they consider less risky to buy conventionally grown as they tend to be less heavily sprayed.

Just because a food is on the clean fifteen doesn't make buying its superior, organic counterpart a bad idea! I recommend always buying organic wherever and whenever possible.

The next time you're at the grocery store, make an effort to spend a little more and safeguard your health by buying these foods organic:

The Dirty Dozen	The Clean Fifteen
Apples	Asparagus
Bell peppers	Avocados
Celery	Cabbage
Cherry tomatoes	Cantaloupe (rock melon)
Collard greens	Eggplant (aubergine)
Cucumbers	Grapefruit
Grapes	Kiwifruit
Hot peppers	Mangoes

The Dirty Dozen	**The Clean Fifteen**
Kale	Mushrooms
Nectarines	Onions
Peaches	Papayas
Potatoes	Peas – frozen
Spinach	Pineapples
Strawberries	Sweet corn
Summer squash	Sweet potatoes

Watching out for Genetically Modified Organisms

When a food doesn't have an organic seal, it may be a genetically modified organism (GMO). Increasingly many foods available in stores are genetically modified (GM), including most papayas and sweet corn, two of the foods on the supposed Clean Fifteen list. The tricky thing is that you can't tell if a food is GM just by looking at it. GM foods have had their DNA altered in some way, with the resulting 'frankenfoods' more closely resembling a science project than real, wholesome food. Although the US government deems these foods safe for human consumption and requires no explicit labeling of them as GMO, I suggest approaching these foods with extreme caution. GMOs are just too new for us to really know any potentially hazardous effects on our health (and of course the environment), but early evidence is pointing towards 'not good'.

Luckily, one way consumers can protect themselves from GMOs is to read the label. You have to pay a little extra attention – which is another great mindfulness practice you can incorporate into your life!

PLU codes are the little stickers stuck on produce in the US and Canada. You may need to remember to bring your glasses with you while grocery shopping, because these stickers are quite small!

Conventionally Grown	**Organically Grown**	**Genetically Modified**
4-digit code	5-digits starting with #9	5-digits starting with #8
Example: Conventionally grown banana: 4011	Example: Organically grown banana: 94011	Example: GMO banana: 84011

Decoding 'organic'

The next time you're shopping for organic foods in North America, look for the USDA Organic seal. As with most product labeling, the wording is specific. Only foods with 95 to 100 percent organic ingredients can use the USDA Organic seal.

100 Percent Organic: Foods that are made with 100 percent organic ingredients.

Organic: Foods that contain at least 95 percent organic ingredients.

Made with organic ingredients: Foods that contain at least 70 percent organic ingredients may list specific organic ingredients on the front of the package, but they cannot use the USDA organic seal.

Contains organic ingredients: Foods that contain less than 70 percent organic ingredients may list specific organic ingredients on the information panel of the package, but they cannot use the organic seal.

Buyer Beware: Buying Food

Considering the 20,000 new products that hit the shelves every year, on top of all the conflicting information about what's healthy and what's not, it's no wonder that you can get confused about what to eat. In today's overloaded and complex food environment, knowing how to make the healthiest choices for you and your family is becoming increasingly challenging.

With all the guidelines offered in this chapter, you now have a good foundation to help you navigate your way when buying food – whether it's in restaurants, grocery stores or even health food stores. In this last section I look at a few more tips for visiting the grocery store and suggest a few alternative solutions to grocery shopping.

Mindful grocery shopping

Two places that have a large influence on your health and your mindful eating journey are your kitchen and the grocery store. Your kitchen is only as supportive as the stock it holds, and how you choose to stock it depends on how you navigate the grocery store (see the later section 'Exploring your alternatives to the supermarket' for some great ideas on other places to source your food).

If one of your primary objectives in eating more mindfully is to establish a healthier relationship with food, then maintaining a healthy kitchen is a great place to start. (Chapter 4 has information on establishing mindful eating goals.) A healthy kitchen relies on stocking it with the good stuff, which involves being a smart grocery shopper and discovering how to master the maze of products and avoid all the traps and distractions of cheap junk food that you'd rather not take home with you.

The next time you go grocery shopping try to follow these key helpful tips to stocking a healthy kitchen:

✓ **Shop the periphery of the grocery store:** The periphery is where all the real food hangs out. The middle aisles are where the packaged, highly processed food is.

✓ **Stick mostly to the produce section and spend most of your time here:** People tend to repeatedly buy the same things, so try something new and buy a wide variety of fresh fruits and vegetables. Try to eat the colors of the rainbow and intuitively pick the colors that are currently singing to you. Select organic produce if they stock it. If your grocery store doesn't carry any organic produce, find out where your local health food store is and see what organic produce they sell there.

✓ **Avoid grocery shopping on an empty stomach:** Low blood sugar can wreak havoc on anyone's plan to eat more healthfully. Have a healthy snack before you go food shopping.

✓ **Work with a shopping list:** Besides being a great way to stay organized, working with a shopping list discourages you from impulsively buying foods that are cleverly placed to entice you into temptation.

✓ **Try to avoid buying packaged foods:** Think about setting this as one of your mindful eating goals and aim to go one week (or even one day!) without eating anything from a package. If you're considering a packaged food item at the store, try to avoid products:

- That have a long list of ingredients.
- That have ingredients you don't recognize.
- With soy, corn, wheat and sugar (and all of their myriad forms and hidden names).
- That contain cheap oils like soybean, canola or vegetable oils.
- With trans fats.
- With a high sodium content.

✓ **Avoid buying packaged foods in bulk:** Getting a good deal feels great, and you save a little money, but what about what you're *gaining* – like all the extra pounds from mindlessly eating more food out of a bigger package. You may think, 'Not me! I don't do that!' But guess what? Everyone does it. People eat more from large packages, serving containers and off bigger plates without being aware of it – mindless eating again! Skip the huge multipack crackers and cereals. Even the visual cue of seeing those packages at home entices you to eat more, more often. If you just can't help yourself, try storing the big boxes out of sight, like in a sealed, safe place in the garage and only bring out small packages at a time, even if you have to repackage the contents yourself.

Exploring your alternatives to the supermarket

The modern food system is set up in a way so that you can go to one place to buy all your food – the grocery store. Although it provides more convenience for you, the grocery store also contributes to the greater disconnect and separation from your food source.

Today, new food-buying alternatives are popping up and helping close that gap, providing healthy whole-food solutions for people.

Farmers' markets

Farmers' markets are emerging all over the place, becoming more of a mainstream solution to buying food in cities all over the world. Farmers' markets are usually full of organic, fresh, local and vibrantly colorful produce, not to mention local artisan products. With a focus on sustainability, farmers' markets tend to attract people with a health-conscious focus on whole foods.

Farmers' markets are great places to connect with and support local farmers and ask them about their farming practices. Making friends with the people who grow your food can prove to be a very special connection. If it interests you, ask if you can take a tour of their farms, and if you really like what they're growing, ask if you can arrange a weekly pickup from them and also let them know you're always willing to take excess produce off their hands!

If you live in a cold climate, one way to increase your year-round intake of whole foods is to buy produce in bulk when it's in abundance and freeze it for the winter months. Most fruits, like peaches, pears and all the berry varieties, freeze really well. Some other ideas include buying basil in bulk, making pesto and freezing it. Fresh pressed apple juice also does great in the freezer, and so do peas and corn off the cob.

Join a produce delivery service

As the demand increases for local, organic produce, wonderfully organized organic food distribution services like CSA (community supported agriculture) or vegetable box schemes are sprouting up in cities all over the world to provide city residents access to fresh, high-quality produce. Some of these programs include drop-off services and some provide a specific location and allocate a certain day for pick-ups.

When you become member of a CSA, for example, you typically buy a share for an entire season of produce, usually upfront. This initial payment supports the local farmer to plan for the season, invest in farm equipment, make repairs or purchase new seeds. Your weekly produce box offers a variety of produce that changes as the season progresses. By supporting your local farmer, everyone wins.

Join a food co-operative

Another option you can look into is food co-operatives, also called co-ops. Typically, food co-ops focus on local organic foods, and after you become a member, you receive better prices on the foods you buy, saving you money on your weekly grocery bills. The other good part about food co-ops is that decisions on how the co-op is run are decided by its members – now that's food empowerment!

Chapter 7

Mindful Meal Preparation

- -

In This Chapter

▶ Exploring your kitchen as a healing sanctuary

▶ Discovering how to detoxify your kitchen

▶ Approaching meal preparation with creative flair

- -

*O*ne of the primary purposes of mindful eating is to foster a healthy relationship with food. This means taking into account the consequences of your food choices on your health.

Since mindful eating encompasses the time before and after meals, it includes the mindful preparation of your meals – preparing and eating whole, organic foods as much as possible and limiting time spent eating out at restaurants.

The kitchen was once the focal point of the house, and people devoted a lot more time to making and preparing meals from scratch. In this chapter explore how you can get reacquainted with your kitchen and set it up to support you and your mindful eating goals.

Exploring Your Relationship with Your Kitchen

Let's face it, in today's reality, you may not have the time (or don't want to make the time) to feed yourself healthfully.

Take a moment to reflect on what your current relationship is to cooking (or non-cooking, for all you raw foodies out there!). Do you view preparing meals as a chore? Are you tired of it?

Feel like you're running out of ideas? Intimidated or over-whelmed by the thought of trying to make new meals?

Now, imagine yourself in the kitchen about to make a meal. What do you feel? Bored? Nervous? Stressed out? Responsible for others health and well-being? Excited to experiment and explore? Do you feel calm and at peace or are you stricken with guilt, shame or anxiety when you're in your kitchen?

If you have a lot of negative associations when thinking about your relationship to your kitchen, don't feel bad about it! (Feeling bad never helps anyway.) For many people, the kitchen has become another workplace, and making meals has become another item to cross off the daily to-do list, especially if you are feeding a family, work-ing a full time job and feeling the pressure to come up with a range of meals creative and delicious enough to keep every-one healthy and happy.

If this rings true for you, mindfulness is the antidote to what-ever challenging experience you are having in the kitchen – even if all you need is to brush up on your rusty kitchen skills! In which case, see the related sidebar, 'Getting creative with food' for some helpful ideas.

Getting creative with food

In addition to practicing mindful-ness in the kitchen, you may want to improve your culinary skills. Here are some ideas to help get you started:

✔ Take a cooking class.

✔ Watch cooking shows – and be mindful of which ones! Many cooking programs showcase very unhealthy foods.

✔ Take a health-themed food vacation.

✔ Buy a new cookbook (there are thousands to choose from!).

✔ Take an online course.

✔ Watch how-to recipe videos on YouTube.

✔ Start a recipe swap with friends or your mindful eating social support group.

✔ Take a culinary class that teaches proper knife skills.

Getting a fresh perspective on your kitchen

The practice of mindfulness helps reduce anxiety and stress, ease depression, smooth out fluctuating moods and emotions and increase happiness – all from simply paying attention!

You can take this mindfulness practice and apply it to meal preparation in the kitchen and transform it into joyful time spent alone, with friends or with your family (Chapter 10 has more on mindful eating for families).

If you've noticed yourself falling into mindless habits in the kitchen or have a strong resistance to preparing your own meals, I'd like to offer an alternative perspective and invite you to see your kitchen – and the time you spend making meals in it – through new eyes.

Your kitchen is a very special place. It's where you co-create and collaborate with the abundance from nature to nourish your body, mind and spirit. Your kitchen is the primary place where you can affirm the healthy visions of your life by preparing whole foods to sustain your life and also perhaps the lives of your most precious loved ones. It's where you can align and tap into your most profound and potent source of healing – your food source.

The kitchen can be your sanctuary, where you find peace of mind, breathe more deeply, relax into yourself, rejuvenate your spirit and take delight in the simple pleasures of life. It's a sacred place where you can sing, laugh, connect with nature, spend time with loved ones, learn, heal and . . . practice mindfulness!

Seeing your kitchen as a sanctuary allows you to view your time spent there as a meaningful, joyful and integral part of your life. Adopting a positive association with your kitchen enables you to slow down and become present for this special, life-sustaining gift of meal creation. When you become present, the simple act of peeling a carrot or washing an apple is a truly amazing experience as you surrender to the awe of the absolute miracle of life!

Think of your kitchen as your playground or artist's studio and remind yourself to be playful and have fun! It's a place where magic happens – where alchemy is performed to create food combinations that sing to your soul.

Expressing love is one of the most profound ways you express your gratitude. Your kitchen is a place where you can express your love – love for your family, love for yourself, love for your body, love for your life and love for nature.

Stepping into the kitchen: Mindful transitioning

How often do you notice your daily stresses spilling into the kitchen with you? When you have a lot on your plate, snapping out of it and into a good mood to become more calm, grounded and graceful in the kitchen is often hard. But trying to shake off any irritation, grudges, tensions and negative feelings before entering your kitchen is important. A ritualized routine for transitioning into the kitchen and getting ready to prepare a meal can help you connect to your underlying intentions, inherent wisdom and mindful attention to the present moment.

Although not backed by science, some people say, 'Our mood affects the food,' so how about leaving your emotional baggage at the door? This habit is a great way to practice letting go and starting to associate your kitchen with a more positive mental mindset. (The later section 'Minding your mood in the kitchen' has more on the importance of your mindset.)

Try placing a handwritten sign saying, 'Leave it at the door' above or next to your kitchen door as a visual reminder for yourself. Taking five minutes to sit down and focus on your breathing before you walk into the kitchen can make a wonderful mindful transition.

Decide to let go of any negative feelings before you step into the kitchen and allow yourself to be guided by your inner creative wisdom. Feeling good allows you to step into the flow of inspired meal creation, mindfully crafting wonderfully delicious meals guided by the flow and grace of the divine creative life-force.

Any time you transition from one activity to another, you may find yourself doing it mindlessly. Any transition offers an excellent opportunity to practice mindfulness and is helpful for grounding yourself in your next activity. After you've prepared the meal, for example, take a moment to take three conscious breaths and pause before you start to eat. After you've finished eating, take another moment to pause and mindfully transition to cleaning up.

Invest in an apron so that you can just go for it in the kitchen without worrying about your clothes getting dirty.

Mindfulness in the kitchen

Maintaining a healthy relationship with food requires a holistic, multi-dimensional approach – it's not just what you eat, but *how* and *why* you eat, as well as how you *relate* to food, eating, your body and even your life that paints the bigger picture of your health and well-being.

Mindful eating and mindful meal preparation are just two of the many ways you can incorporate mindfulness into the fullness of your life. Considering all the benefits that mindful living has to offer, establishing mindfulness in the kitchen (and with food) is a great place to start.

Exploring your mindless kitchen habits

Before thinking about mindfulness in the kitchen, start by looking at all the mindless tendencies and habits that you have already developed in the kitchen. When you become aware of them, you can consciously choose to change them (if you want to!).

What are your most mindless kitchen habits? What do you repeatedly do in the kitchen that you want to change?

Some of the ways you may experience mindlessness in the kitchen are:

- ✔ Rushing to prepare meals or grabbing food from the kitchen to eat on the run.
- ✔ Mindlessly eating with the fridge door open.

✔ Grazing at food on the counter.

✔ Standing up to eat at the counter.

✔ Watching TV while eating in the kitchen.

✔ Talking on the phone while eating.

✔ Not paying attention to cleanliness in the kitchen; leaving dishes unwashed or food out on the counter.

Do any of these ring a bell for you? Do other mindless habits not mentioned here spring to mind?

Establishing mindfulness in the kitchen

So now that you've mindfully transitioned into the kitchen, leaving unnecessary baggage at the door, and you've become more aware of your mindless kitchen habits, the time has come to explore some mindful kitchen ways.

In a culture that is constantly on the go, practicing mindfulness in the kitchen allows you to slow down and enjoy the precious moments in your life.

Start by setting your intention to pay attention and consciously notice what you want to pay attention to.

Knives, kitchen tools with a blade (blenders and food processors), ovens and hot stoves are definitely worth paying careful attention to!

Think of your breath as home base. Simply turning your attention back towards your breath is an excellent mindfulness exercise to start with in the kitchen. If you notice your mind wandering, bring your attention and focus back to your breath and notice how you're breathing. Since you're also likely to be moving in the kitchen, mindfulness of movements also becomes a point of focus, as outlined in the next exercise.

Bring your attention to the movements of your body in the kitchen and notice the sensations that you feel. Mindfulness requires engaging all of your senses. Feel the sensations of holding a knife and an apple in your hand. What does it feel like? What do you see? What do you smell? What do you hear as you slice into the apple? What emotions or feelings does this conjure up in you? If you're making a fruit salad, use your awareness to engage the full range of sensory experience. Feel your hand opening the fridge door, hear the water as you turn on the tap, notice the colors of the food.

You can also use mindfulness in the kitchen to become aware of and notice what it is your body wants for nourishment.

Minding your mood in the kitchen

One of the most profound changes that you can make in your kitchen is to simply shift your attitude and embrace the time that you spend preparing food in it with mindfulness and respect for the delightful and sacred activity that it is, and honor the sacred space that you get to do it in. If you fall into the habit of viewing your time in the kitchen as a monotonous, mundane chore, you disconnect from the specialness of the food that you are preparing for your body. And if you harbor resentment while preparing food, you may be directly infusing your food with negative emotions.

Raising the vibes

The next time you're making a meal in the kitchen stop and check your mood around the food. What you choose to focus on is what you will see manifest in your life!

Some ways that you can raise the vibes in the kitchen are:

- ✔ **Playing music while you prepare food or clean up:** Choose your music wisely; select positive, up-lifting and inspiring music. Music has the power to boost your mood in an instant, but if music is going to potentially distract you from being mindful of preparing your meal, then consider skipping this option. My best advice: experiment and see what works for you!

- ✔ **Practicing an attitude of gratitude:** Mindful meal preparation embodies a sense of connectedness with your food source. The real secret is to stay in awe of the miracle of food and to foster an attitude of gratitude and total reverence for the divine forces of nature. Chapters 5 and 8 have more on fostering gratitude.

✔ **Setting an intention:** A powerful way to align with your deepest values is to start your meal preparation by setting a heartfelt intention. Setting an intention is also a great way to instantly shift from viewing something as mundane and repetitive to viewing it as sacred or special. For instance:

'May the food I prepare carry the vibration of love into my body and those who I am feeding.'

✔ **Setting an aspiration:** An aspiration is like setting an affirmation, but it can have a far greater reach – extending out to all sentient beings. This is an easy, powerful and effective way to stay and feel connected to the rest of humanity. Examples are:

'May all beings be free from hunger.'

'May all beings feel loved and nourished.'

Lowering the stress

Many of the sources of stress in your life, such as your job, the stock market, relationships and the never-ending to-do lists, are perceived stresses (which doesn't make them any less real!). They are only as real and stressful as you perceive them to be. Mindfulness is a wonderful antidote to the everyday stresses you feel, and mindful meal preparation can play a wonderful part, too. Practicing mindful meal preparation reminds you to connect with what's actually real, right in front of you – food, hands, sink, water, cutting board – and encourages you to have a direct experience with reality.

Feng shui the kitchen

Your outer reality is a reflection of your inner reality, so start here, in your kitchen. Implement the changes that you need to make in your outer environment to feel at peace and at home in your inner environment.

Chaos and disorganization in our outer reality encourage chaos of our inner reality.

According to the dictionary, *feng shui* directly translates to 'wind-water' in English. Feng shui is a Chinese system governing the arrangement and orientation of buildings and objects to harmonize the human experience with the surrounding environment and the flow of energy (*qi*).

A natural way to clean

Many of the household cleaners sold today are quite toxic. You can easily make yourself a homemade cleaner that is inexpensive, works excellently and smells great!

Here's one particular recipe that you can use for all cleaning purposes, including cleaning floors, counter-tops and sinks:

✔ Get an empty spray bottle and fill it about two-thirds full with water.

✔ Add a splash of regular vinegar.

✔ Add about a dozen drops of lemon or peppermint oil.

✔ Add about a dozen drops and oregano oil.

✔ Add about a dozen drops of grape seed extract.

This is just one household cleaning recipe that you can use. A simple search online will render many more!

You can use the principals of feng shui to set up an environment that is supportive of your mindful eating lifestyle. Operating in a clean, organized space helps you to navigate the kitchen more mindfully – not to mention more efficiently and more gracefully!

Keep things clean and orderly out of respect for the space that you are creating in and for what you're creating with! Fine-tune your kitchen so that the energy flows effortlessly and allows you to feel more at ease in your space.

Detoxifying your kitchen

Before thinking about detoxifying your diet, you first need to start with detoxifying your kitchen. Now is an excellent time to clear out the clutter!

When was the last time you cleaned out your kitchen? Here are some tips to help support you on your mindful eating journey:

✔ Clear out all the foods in your pantry. Place all the foods on your kitchen table and wipe down the shelves with a cleaner (see the nearby sidebar, 'A natural way to clean' on using a natural household cleaner). Go through each food item and ask yourself if this food is supporting or hindering your journey towards vibrant health. Consider removing processed foods, canned foods that contain preservatives, foods with a long list of ingredients or ingredients that you don't recognize, and foods that have been there for over a year.

✔ Remove all food that has passed the expiry date!

✔ Make a list of your most addictive foods, the foods that you struggle with the most and find hard to stop eating after you start. Consider discarding these foods or storing them in a less prominent place in your kitchen so that they are not regularly in your line of sight to help prevent constant triggers; remember the saying, 'Out of sight, out of mind.' You can leave these foods there and find out how to eat small amounts of them mindfully if you decide to discover your middle-way approach (flip back to Chapter 4 for more about the middle-way approach).

✔ Do the same with your fridge. Empty the entire fridge and wipe it down. Throw away all outdated foods, leftovers hidden in the back of the fridge and foods that you no longer wish to consume. Restock it with the types of whole foods outlined in Chapter 6 – predominantly fresh fruits and vegetables!

✔ Clear your most frequently used counter space.

✔ Clear out distractions like a TV.

✔ Say goodbye to outdated kitchen equipment (what have you not touched in the past five years?). But before you give it away, ask yourself if you can start using it to help support your whole-foods lifestyle.

✔ Throw away broken or worn tools you no longer use.

✔ Clean out junk drawers and organize them in a way that supports you. Maybe you can allocate a drawer to your mindful eating journey and stock it with loose-leaf paper and pens for recipe ideas.

✔ Make space for a recipe binder and start collecting recipes you'd like to try.

✔ Place a magnetic shopping pad on your fridge so you can keep an ongoing grocery list to make grocery shopping day as easy as pie.

Keep it organized

Now that you have some new space available, organize the kitchen items you have left in an efficient way. Make room for your blender on your counter to encourage you to make smoothies on a daily basis (check out the great smoothie recipes in the minitable nearby) and put away other countertop items you use less often – like your microwave.

Ask yourself if you feel calmer when you're in an orderly environment. Or even one that just looks more orderly. What strategies work for you to keep things looking uncluttered and organized?

Mindful Meal Creation

Preparing meals at home gives you greater control over the freshness of the food you use and the quality of the ingredients. You also avoid food colorings, chemicals, food additives and other unnecessary items.

Smart food preparation starts with high quality ingredients. Head to Chapter 6 for guidelines on choosing healthy foods mindfully.

A drop of inspiration: Recipe exploration

Try not to buy food products that you can easily make at home. Adopt the attitude that the meals you're going to make will be better than anything you can buy in the store! Listed below are just a few recipe ideas to get your mind thinking in the right direction: towards healthy whole foods.

Bring the energy of playfulness into the kitchen with you. Even if you're following recipes, try considering the recipe as a guideline only and then create your own version of it.

Smooth over your morning with smoothies

If you grab a coffee and muffin or bagel on your way to work every morning to save time, look no further. Preparing breakfast doesn't get much easier than making a morning smoothie. Smoothies are a great way to get more fruits and vegetables into your diet. They are easy to make and convenient to clean up after. In the past few years, an enormous smoothie revolution has taken place, and you can now find countless smoothie recipes to suit any taste.

Here are a couple of smoothie ideas. All you need is a high-powered blender for these smoothie recipes. Wash all ingredients (unless frozen) beforehand. In these smoothie recipes you can add as much or as little water as you like. If you're using frozen ingredients (especially frozen bananas), the less water you add, the more your smoothie will resemble ice cream.

If you use water, try to use pure, filtered water. If you have access to coconuts, you can add coconut water instead of water. As usual, use organic ingredients whenever possible and experiment with any combination you can think of – the options are limitless!

Blend at high speed until smooth and creamy. Serve and enjoy.

Pear-Cilantro (Coriander) Smoothie	*Cucumber-Banana Smoothie*	*Blueberry-Spinach Smoothie*
2 pears, cut up and inner core removed	1 medium cucumber	½ cup blueberries
1 bunch of cilantro (coriander)	1 bunch of mint	3 bananas, peeled
3 bananas (fresh or frozen), peeled	3 bananas, peeled	1 handful of spinach
1 or 2 dates	2 dates	

Food for thought: Lunch and dinner recipe ideas

Looking for some new ideas for lunch or dinner? Try some of
these suggestions.

Quinoa Tabbouleh Salad

Quinoa's delicious taste and delicate, soft texture have made
it a popular substitute for starchier pasta, potatoes and rice.
It's high in a wide range of amino acids (an excellent protein
source) and a number of minerals, including phosphorus,
magnesium, manganese and iron.

1. Measure out 1 cup of any variety of quinoa you like
   and rinse thoroughly.

2. Place it in a pan with 2 cups of water, cover and bring
   it to the boil. Reduce heat and let it cook for another
   10 to15 minutes. (Make sure not to overcook the
   quinoa or it tastes stickier and starchier than normal.
   You also don't want it to be crunchy, but light and
   fluffy.)

3. Place cooked quinoa in a bowl and let it cool down
   before placing it in the fridge.

While the quinoa is cooling off, wash and dice up a cucumber
and three medium-sized tomatoes into medium-sized cubes.
Chop up a bunch of parsley and mix everything together
with the quinoa. Top with the Creamy Ginger Lemon Honey
Dressing described later or drizzle a teaspoonful of flaxseed
oil on top with a squeeze of fresh lemon and sprinkle with
cumin to taste.

As you prepare meals, be guided by your intuition. If you feel
pulled to add a certain spice that you don't normally add, give
it a try!

Roast Pumpkin (Winter Squash)

If you live in a cold climate and only have access to fresh local
and organic foods for part of the year, a great way to up your
intake of these nutritious foods is to buy certain foods in bulk
to store for the winter months. If kept in a cool, dry space,
pumpkin stores exceptionally well for three to five months.

1. Preheat oven to 375 degrees Fahrenheit (190 degrees Celsius).

2. Cut pumpkin in half (use your muscles!).

3. Scoop out pumpkin seeds (although you can roast those too if you like, in a separate pan).

4. Place the pumpkin halves face down on a lightly oiled baking sheet (coconut oil is excellent for withstanding high heat).

5. The cooking time is flexible, usually about 45 minutes. Cook until the inner pumpkin is tender enough to easily poke it with a fork through the skin.

Eat this pumpkin mashed (try it with a drizzle of Creamy Ginger Lemon Honey Dressing described later) or use it as the base of a pumpkin soup.

Steamed Asparagus

Nothing tastes quite like freshly picked asparagus. I assure you, it's quite different from even one-week-old store-bought asparagus. When it's fresh, as with all fresh veggies, it's bursting with juice and is a lot more flavorful. When asparagus is in season in your local area, eat it raw with a dip or try simple steamed asparagus as a side dish, or even as a main!

1. Place water in the bottom half of a steamer-pan set and turn on the stove to high heat.

2. Wash and trim one bunch of asparagus (although you don't need to trim the ends if the asparagus is super fresh!).

3. Place the asparagus in the top half of the steamer-pan set and cover with a lid.

4. Bring the water to the boil and steam the asparagus for three to five minutes, depending on the thickness of the asparagus, or until asparagus is tender. Avoid over-steaming.

5. Remove lid and drain.

Add a squeeze of lemon juice for an added zesty flavor.

Beet (Beetroot) Dip

Wash all ingredients and place in a high-powered blender or food processor:

> 1 medium beet (beetroot), roughly chopped up – no need to peel!
>
> ½ apple, roughly chopped up
>
> 1½ stalks of celery
>
> 1 medium avocado, peeled and pit removed
>
> Juice from 1 or 2 small lemons, to taste
>
> 1 tablespoon mixed Italian seasoning

Blend together until smooth and serve as a dip for vegetables, a side to a main meal or as a thick salad dressing.

Creamy Ginger Lemon Honey Dressing

In a blender place:

> ¾ cup of coconut water or regular water
>
> ½ cup of organic raw tahini
>
> ¼ cup of fresh lemon juice
>
> 1-inch (3-cm) knob of ginger, peeled
>
> 2 teaspoons ground cumin
>
> 1 clove of garlic (optional)
>
> 1 tablespoon honey (or another whole food sweetener, like 2 dates)

Blend at high speed until creamy. Chill for 30 minutes before serving on top of a green leaf salad, roast vegetables or on top of Quinoa Tabbouleh Salad (see the earlier recipe).

Mindful food preparation: Bring out your good china

Since you just went through all the (mindful) effort to make delicious food, try to pay a little extra attention to your food presentation.

Pick an evening to prepare a themed meal and set your table to reflect this theme. For example, make a Mexican fiesta or Italian themed night and get creative with your dinner setting.

Even if you're eating alone, make it special and visually appealing; drink your water out of a wine glass, use beautiful or colorful tableware that brings a smile to your face. Whatever makes you feel satisfied with the way your meal looks – try it!

Part III
Practicing Mindful Eating

Top five ways to become a mindful eating pro

🖊 **Strengthen the direct line of communication with your inner body awareness:** a whole universe exists within you and after you start to explore that and keep a direct line of open communication between body and mind, you're guided towards what and how much to eat. But you need to listen and pay attention to receive the message!

🖊 **Discover how to do a quick body scan before you eat:** this can help you receive the valuable information that your body has to offer you. Chapter 8 has a guided body-scan practice for you.

🖊 **Get into the habit of slowing down:** it's harder to pay attention when you're rushing around. Slowing down is a practice that is conducive to fostering mindfulness.

🖊 **Approach food with curiosity and playfulness:** You can play many different games and exercises to practice and explore mindful eating. Adopt a beginner's mind and have fun with them!

🖊 **Explore food with the full range of your senses:** the act of eating has much to offer you in the way of pleasurable sensory experience, but only if you're present enough to experience it.

web extras

Find four simple ways to get started with mindful eating at www.dummies.com/extras/mindfuleating.

In this part . . .

- ✔ Dive into exploring the many different practical applications of mindfulness before, during and after you eat.

- ✔ Understand how to practice the body scan and use the hunger-fullness scale to support mindful inner-body awareness.

- ✔ Discover how to slow down, press the mute button and give thanks.

- ✔ Find out how to mindfully explore the full range of your senses while you eat.

Chapter 8

Tooling Up for Mindful Eating

· ·

In This Chapter

▶ Exploring your body from the inside out with the body scan

▶ Finding out how to tune into hunger and fullness levels

▶ Avoiding distractions whilst eating

▶ Discovering the benefits of slowing down your eating habits

· ·

*I*magine that you have a mindful eating tool belt and each tool represents a different skill that you can draw upon. In this chapter you'll become familiar with five very handy mindful eating tools that you can practice and utilize in any situation. Cultivating the following five skills helps you on your path to eating more mindfully:

✓ Practicing a body scan

✓ Tuning into your hunger with the hunger-fullness scale

✓ Eating without distraction

✓ Giving thanks

✓ Slowing down

The first two skills are related to inner body awareness. When you practice and become familiar with the body scan, you can implement a shorter version of it before meals, which naturally leads you into hunger and fullness exploration.

After you've tuned into your inner body awareness, with the third skill, you shift your focus to your external environment and modify your habitual patterns of distraction to simply concentrate on your eating when you eat. The fourth skill – giving thanks – is more of a ritual, and you can draw upon it to set a positive tone for the meal. Slowing down, the fifth skill, also encourages you to adopt new behavioral patterns around eating as you teach yourself to slow down, which goes hand in hand with mindfulness.

You can use these five tools in any combination. However, this order offers you a natural progression from starting to finishing a meal. You may also want to combine them with the formal mindful eating practices outlined in Chapter 9, or any of the other mindful eating tools offered throughout this book.

Connecting with Your Inner Body

You probably tend to look outside of yourself for answers to the problems that you're seeking to remedy. However, mindfulness offers an inside-out approach. When you become mindful of your thoughts and what you're feeling, both emotionally and physically, you cultivate a natural capacity to care for yourself and you discover how to find greater balance, peace and ease within yourself.

On this journey of mindfulness, *you* are actually the one leading the way. I'm here to support you with knowledge and offer you suggestions of possible paths you can discover and *experience* for yourself. However, the power to make decisions rests in your own hands, as it always has.

Mindfulness offers you a way to connect with your natural body wisdom and guides you on your own path – one that feels the best and makes the most sense to you.

Using the body scan, as well as the hunger-fullness scale, strengthens your natural capacity to tune in to your inner body awareness, helping you to navigate your way to a healthier relationship with food.

Performing a body scan

The body scan is a procedure that involves you lying down and mentally scanning your body, typically from your toes to the top of your head, with a loving attitude towards whatever you're experiencing.

The purpose of the body scan is to cultivate self-awareness, one of the key components of mindfulness. It allows you to gain awareness of your thoughts and the physical sensations of your body – in a sense, feeling it and connecting to your body from the inside out. By taking the time to simply scan your body with your awareness, you strengthen your connection between mind and body.

 Like many mindfulness practices, the body scan's a practice in acceptance – accepting whatever you feel without judging it or trying to change it. It's also a practice in letting go of the need to control what the experience is and simply embracing whatever it is you feel.

Allocating time

For this practice, try to set aside at least 30 to 45 minutes of undisturbed time. Turn off your phone, place a Do Not Disturb sign on your door – whatever you have to do to take this uninterrupted time for yourself. This time is for self-care, rest, relaxation and healing and is a wonderful addition to any stress-reduction program.

Preparing to get comfortable

Being as comfortable as possible is important while practicing the body scan. Follow this quick checklist to help you ease into this practice and avoid disturbances.

- ✔ Before starting, you may want to use the washroom or get a drink of water.
- ✔ Body temperature often drops when you are lying still. Make sure that you're warm during this practice; get a blanket or put on a sweater if you need to.
- ✔ Find a comfortable place to lie down on a flat, level surface. You may want to lie on a carpet or bed or place a cushioned mat on the floor.
- ✔ If you have any problems with your lower back, place a pillow under your knees.
- ✔ If you wear glasses, consider removing them, as you will be closing your eyes.
- ✔ Remove your hair tie if you're wearing one to help your scalp and head relax.
- ✔ Wear loose or comfortable clothing.

Setting your intention

Before you start this practice, set your intention to remain open to whatever you experience. Embracing fully an unpleasant or painful sensation in your body with curiosity and friendliness rather than trying to resist it and move away from it can seem like a radical concept. However, surrendering to a sensation, even if it is pain, is a major step towards acceptance and release of control over the present moment.

Practicing the body scan

For the body scan, you may want to invite someone to read the guided instructions to you or read them thoroughly yourself and work through it based on memory. Or if you have a smart phone, you can also read the instructions on the recorder on your phone and play it back to yourself while you're lying down.

The UC San Diego Health Systems website has free downloadable MP3 files for various body scan exercises at: http://health.ucsd.edu/specialties/mindfulness/mbsr/Pages/audio.aspx

If you'd like to put a compassionate spin on your body scan practice, check out the 'Compassionate Body Scan' by Kristin Neff, produced by Sounds True (http://www.soundstrue.com).

1. Lie down on your back with your arms alongside your body, palms facing up. Elbows are away from your body so your shoulders can relax and your legs are gently spread apart allowing your hips to relax. Your feet are naturally and gently falling open to the sides. Tuck your chin in slightly to elongate the back of your neck. Close your eyes.

2. Focus your attention on your breath. Notice the weight of your body touching the ground. With each exhalation, sink deeper into the mat or floor, letting go of any tension in your body.

   Rest with your awareness on your breath for a few minutes. Notice the rise and fall of your belly or the sensation of air flowing into and out of your nostrils.

3. When you feel ready, move your awareness down to your left toes. Start with your big toe and move your way through each of your toes to your little baby toe, noticing any sensations that you're feeling. Zero in on each toe individually and notice any difference in how they feel. Feel all your left toes together now. Notice, without judgment, how they feel. Are they hot or cold? Can you feel their contact with the air, your socks or perhaps a blanket? Imagine your breath coming into your body through your nose and travelling all the way down into your toes, reversing direction on the out-breath. Do you notice any change in sensation?

If you can't feel anything, that's okay. Just notice and bear witness to the lack of feeling or sensation. Remember that energy is always moving. As you continue to observe, notice any shift in sensations. Remain open to all possibilities.

4. Now expand your awareness from your toes into your foot. With your awareness, scan your foot; notice the sole of your foot, the ball of your toe and the more delicate skin on the top part of your foot. Notice the contact that your heel is making with the ground. Pay attention to sensations in your ankle. Observe what your foot feels like. Again, breathe into the whole left foot, completely relaxing the foot, then letting it go and continuing with your awareness up your leg.

5. Continue to expand your awareness up your leg with curiosity and openness. Go through your calf, your shin, your thigh and hamstring, both the front, back and sides of your leg until you reach your left hip.

6. Move your awareness from your left hip down to your right toes and proceed with the same instructions on your right toes, foot, lower leg and upper leg, up to your right hip.

Notice if your right leg feels different than your left leg.

7. With a gentle, loving attitude, explore your hip area, pelvis, buttocks and all the delicate organs that reside in this area. Notice your lower back and any tension you may be holding there. Breathing into each part, imagine you are breathing new life into this area of your body.

Notice any emotions that come up for you and welcome them in with love, acceptance and a non-judgmental attitude. Notice if you have an impulse to resist or move away from any emotion presenting itself.

8. Move your awareness into your lower torso. In your mind's eye, imagine all the incredible workings of your digestive organs. Every time you eat, they have to work so hard to process, assimilate, filter, detoxify and cleanse for you, supporting the health of your body and your life. Notice your belly inflating as you breathe in and notice how it feels when you breathe out and your belly deflates. Notice the feeling of your back against the floor. What sensations can you detect? Breathe into each part of this area of your body, slowly releasing the breath each time.

9. Bring your awareness up to your chest and upper back. Witness the power of your heart's beat. Notice any tightness you may be holding on to in your chest, upper back and shoulders. Notice your lungs fill up with air and what that sensation feels like.

10. Then move your awareness to your fingers on both hands, scanning with your awareness up both arms at the same time. Work through your fingers, hands, wrists, forearms, upper arms and into your shoulders. Explore each body part slowly, breathing into it and then gradually moving on, paying attention to what you're feeling in each area.

11. Bring your awareness to your neck and move up into your jaw. Notice if you're holding any tightness in your jaw and your face. Notice your cheeks, your lips, your nose and eyes. Notice your forehead and observe if it's scrunched up or furrowed. Allow the muscles in your head and face to relax as you breathe into them, opening up to any physical or emotional sensations that present themselves to you in this moment. Reflect on the incredible power of your brain and your capacity to have awareness and be conscious.

12. From here, bring your awareness to your entire body as one unified field of energy and breathe into your body as a whole.

    Continue to allow your breath to feed your body with oxygen, nourishing each of your cells with renewed life.

13. Thank yourself for taking the time to nourish your mind, body and spirit in this way. Rest in this stillness for as long as you need.

14. When you're ready to get up, change your position slowly by first turning over onto your side and resting there for as long as you need. Slowly prop yourself up on your side and bring yourself to a sitting position. Allow yourself to ease into whatever you need to do next, taking your time and maintaining a level of inner body awareness for as long as possible, especially if you're going to be eating a snack or a meal.

Although the body scan is typically a lying-down practice and can take 30 to 45 minutes, you can also implement it while in sitting meditation or do a relatively quick scan of the body while sitting in a chair before a meal, using this exercise as a way to tune into your hunger and fullness level, which I outline in the next section.

Exploring the Hunger-fullness Scale

In western culture's over-abundant food environment, most people in developed countries don't experience true hunger on a daily basis. When you feel the slightest level of discomfort you can all to o easily remedy that feeling with food – after all, you're biologically designed to seek out food for your survival, and you wouldn't last very long without it. But how often do you eat when you're barely hungry at all?

As I discussed in Chapter 3, you're influenced by many undetected cues that habitually drive you to eat when you're not hungry. You eat based on other people, the time of day, how you feel, the weather; all of these factors influence when and how much you eat. Many people confess to me that they don't know when they should eat, and they also don't know when to stop after they've started.

By assigning your hunger (and then subsequently your fullness) a number on a scale from 1 to 10, with 1 being the most hungry and 10 being the most full, you encourage yourself to check and evaluate your relative hunger and fullness, giving yourself an inner navigational guide to eating.

Look at the Figure 8-1 for guidance on the hunger-fullness scale.

1	2	3	4	5	6	7	8	9	10
Very Hungry		Hungry			Neutral	Comfortably Full			Stuffed

Figure 8-1: Use the hunger-fullness scale to work out just how hungry you really are.

1. **Before a meal:** Evaluate your hunger level. How hungry are you feeling? Are you in the 1 to 4 hunger range? What physical sensations are indicating that you're hungry? Are you feeling tired, faint or weak? Where do you feel hungry? Place your hand on the part of your body you feel your hunger is coming from. Is it your belly, your mouth, your throat, your heart or your mind?

2. **During a meal:** When you have completed about half of your meal, take a moment to pause and put down your eating utensils. Check yourself again. Where are you on the scale now? Are you in the 5 to 7 range or are you rapidly approaching the Full range above 7? How do you feel about stopping eating the meal at this point? Notice what leaving food on your plate would feel like. Do you feel guilty? Could you save it for later? How do you think you'll feel if you continue to eat past this point? Do you think you'll regret it? Will you feel uncomfortably full? If you decide to continue to eat, eat as slowly and mindfully as possible, checking in periodically from here.

3. **After a meal:** When you have decided to stop eating, notice where you are on the scale. Are you a comfortably full 7 to 8 or are you painfully full at 9 or 10? Have you unbuttoned your jeans by this point? Are you still hungry for another serving of food? If you're contemplating getting up for more food, take five minutes to let your stomach settle and then check in with your hunger levels again.

Any time after you finish a meal where you incorporated the hunger-fullness scale, turn to your mindful eating journal and make comments or notes about what you discovered. (Flip to Chapter 4 for more on starting a mindful eating journal.) Jot down how it felt to eat until you were comfortably full or how it felt to eat until you were stuffed. Ask yourself how you feel after this experience and what you can do differently or repeat next time so that you feel at peace and at ease after your meal.

Awareness, in and of itself, helps support change. Just because you evaluate your hunger and notice you're not hungry doesn't mean that you're not allowed to eat.

This book is not about restriction and rules. Whether you choose to eat or not is up to you. You may, however, check in and notice that you're not hungry and also note your desire for ice cream in that moment. You may comment, 'That's interesting. I'm not hungry, but my mind wants ice cream right now.' This process is how you discover how to make mindful decisions. You can ask yourself a series of self-inquiring questions, as outlined in Chapter 13, or proceed to eat a bowl of ice cream in a mindful manner, paying attention to each and every bite and how you feel throughout this eating experience, as well as how you feel afterwards. Eating with awareness, whether you're hungry or not, is an excellent step in the right direction. And proceeding to eat mindfully when you're not hungry can offer you valuable insights that affect your future decisions around eating and help you establish a more positive and balanced relationship with food.

Pressing the Mute Button: Tuning Out Pesky Distractions

After you tune into your inner reality, you shift focus to your outer environment and the changes you can make in both your surroundings and your behavior and habitual patterns to support a more mindful eating experience.

I recently saw a magnet on my friend's fridge that read *Mom: Master of Multitasking.* Being able to do multiple things simultaneously is highly praised in our culture. Doing only one thing at a time is regarded as 'weak', 'unambitious' or 'slow'. This culture is where 'eating on the run' takes on a whole new meaning; the third most frequent place Americans eat is in the car while driving! However, in Japanese culture, eating while you walk is considered poor manners, despite being very common in American culture. Eating on the run is not a part of Japanese traditional ways. In Japanese culture, one sits down to eat out of respect, and probably for more practical reasons too, like to avoid spilling food on your clothes!

The pace of life is increasing exponentially, resulting in an era of distraction. When you do multiple things simultaneously, your attention is constantly being pulled in different directions. You can't fully pay attention to one thing because you're being distracted by the other things you're trying to do at the same time!

Keeping up with the many hurdles of life is an on-going challenge, and the wonderful world of entertainment provides a useful distraction, whether it's TV shows, movies, video games, the Internet, shopping or eating out.

If you struggle with your relationship with food, the very first thing you can do to improve that relationship is to remove distractions and concentrate on your eating when you eat. Like in any healthy relationship, you need to pay attention to who (or what) you're in a relationship with! It may sound simple, but for most people paying attention is actually quite difficult given our strong natural tendency towards distraction.

What's your favorite thing to do when you eat? Is it watching television? How about reading the paper? Checking your emails? Listening to your favorite radio program? Start to pay attention to what else you automatically reach for during your meals and note it in your mindful eating journal.

Applying mindfulness to your meals by removing distractions is one of the foundational ways that you can heal a disordered relationship with food. When you remove as many distractions as possible while you eat, you afford yourself the wonderful gift of food! If you struggle with overeating, this simple practice can allow you to actually enjoy the food you're seeking pleasure and satisfaction from. You give yourself permission to enjoy whatever food you have before you and prevent any feelings of guilt, obsession and shame that you may have around food.

Try these tips to tune out distractions while you eat:

- ✔ Try to find a calm, relaxing environment to eat your meal in.

- ✔ If you are at home, make sure the TV, radio and computer are off.

- ✔ Put your cell phone on silent and don't bring your phone to the dining table with you. Remind yourself that you can always check messages after you eat.

- ✔ Clear any newspapers, books or magazines from the table where you're eating to prevent distractions.

- ✔ If you're eating with others, pay extra attention to the potential for being distracted by conversation. Notice if eating and listening at the same time is challenging. Try to avoid talking while eating and focus on one or the other.

- ✔ If you're at work and you feel pressured for time, make an effort to avoid eating at your desk. If you must eat there, at least turn off your computer while you're eating. Try to find a nearby table, preferably outside, and give yourself *at least* 15 minutes to take a lunch break. Although you often don't think you have time, in the long run, taking short breaks actually makes you more productive.

Some things you can control (turning off the TV) and other things you can't (a barking dog outside). While you can't exactly shut out the outside world around you when you eat, you can consciously choose to do only one thing at a time: *when you eat, simply eat.*

Try to eat at least one distraction-free meal per day. Use your mindful eating journal to explore what this experience is like for you. Explore these questions around this experience:

- ✔ Do you notice you gain more or less pleasure from eating when you eat without distraction?

- ✔ Do you feel more or less satisfied after you eat?

- ✔ Do you notice your mind wanders despite having minimal distractions?

- ✔ Is it challenging for you to only eat when you eat? Why do you think that may be?

✔ What does it feel like to eat without distractions? Do you feel bored? More fulfilled? More tuned in to your body's level of hunger and fullness?

If you have a family with children, instilling this mindful eating habit at as young an age as possible is a good idea. Make it a family ritual to turn off the distractions and eat a meal as a family. Teach your children the importance of paying attention to their food and request that they don't bring any distractions to the table. Check out Chapter 10 for more on mindful eating for families.

Giving Thanks: A Speed Bump to Eating

After you've tuned in to your inner body awareness and removed distractions from eating, pause a moment to connect with a feeling of gratitude for the gift of the food before you.

Taking a moment to express and offer gratitude for food has been a customary mealtime ritual in almost all religions and spiritual traditions throughout history, in cultures all over the world.

Some consider giving thanks as a way to bless the food they are about to eat. According to the dictionary, one of the definitions of the word 'bless' means to 'express or feel gratitude toward; to thank'. You can think of giving thanks before the meal as a mealtime blessing or prayer if that resonates for you. If this doesn't align with your belief systems, you can simply think of it as expressing gratitude for the food you eat.

Offering a mealtime blessing doesn't have to be religious, but if you do practice or follow a particular faith, explore what kind of mealtime blessings, prayers or rituals are practiced around food at mealtimes. If your faith has specific quotations relating to meals, consider incorporating them into your eating routine. Only choose what feels in alignment for you. If nothing inspires you, feel free to create your own rituals or blessings!

If you don't follow a particular faith but are spiritually inclined, giving thanks can be a deeply spiritual practice.

Giving thanks for a meal gives you an opportunity to:

- ✔ Acknowledge the importance of food as sustenance for your life.
- ✔ Generate and foster positive feelings of gratitude and appreciation that can influence the health of your mind, body and spirit.
- ✔ Recognize the miracle and divinity of food.
- ✔ Recognize your interconnection with all living beings.
- ✔ Show respect for all life and creation. When you honor food, you also honor yourself and your body.

The many ways to express gratitude

You can give thanks for your food in many ways, and the sky is the limit in terms of how you choose to express your gratitude.

Giving thanks for the elements

You can focus on blessing all or any of the elements that contribute to growing your food, including the rain, the sunshine, the air and the soil – even fire! Millions of microbes and insects, worms and fungi exist in the soil, all of which contribute to making the soil fertile for growing and give the food its nutritive properties. Also, many tiny creatures – bees, flies, wasps, moths and even ants – help to pollinate all the different kinds of flowering plants, including the plants that grow our food.

Giving thanks for the people

Another way you can express gratitude before a meal is to thank all the people who partook in bringing the food before you. This practice is a mindful eating exercise in its own right. You can work backwards or forwards through time, starting with the people in the kitchen who prepared the food or starting with the farmers who picked the food. You can go as far back as thanking the people who planted the seeds. Be creative and make it fun.

Giving thanks for life

You can also take a more spiritually connected approach and tune into the deeper significance of the sustenance that food provides you to live out your life. Here is an example you may want to try or modify:

> I am truly grateful to receive this nourishment from the earth.
>
> I put this food in my body with the highest of intention, to love, support and nourish my being.
>
> May every cell and atom of my being align with and consciously use this vital life force from the earth.
>
> May the energy in this food fuel me on my spiritual journey, so that I can in turn live and carry out my true life's purpose.
>
> May I realize my path of awakening for the benefit of all beings. I infuse this food with love and gratitude.

Getting creative: Different ways to give thanks

You can give thanks when you're alone, silently or out loud, with a group of people or with any number of eating companions. You can invite anyone to say a food blessing, taking turns if you regularly eat with the same people. One person can give thanks or each person can contribute in some small way. If you're eating with a diverse group, explore the different traditions and invite people to share a customary tradition that they're familiar with. You can sing the blessing in a song or you can offer up one or two minutes of silence to allow everyone to connect with their own sense of inner gratitude.

Grab your mindful eating journal and brainstorm some mealtime blessings that feel good for you. Get creative and even make it rhyme if you want to. Maybe you want to write it up and carry it with you or print it out with a nice image to accompany it.

Putting on the Brakes: Discovering How to Slow Down

After you've scanned your body, checked in with your hunger level, removed as many distractions as possible and paused by giving thanks and setting a positive tone for the meal, the next skill to acquire for your tool belt is the art of eating slowly.

Eating slowly can be challenging to do in a culture that's increasingly getting busier and busier – who can possibly afford the time to slow down and enjoy a meal? Yes indeed, everyone's plate is full and overflowing!

Flicking a switch and automatically slowing down when you sit down to eat is really difficult – if you're sitting down to eat at all. You feel as if your mind is still ten steps in front of your body, and that momentum is challenging to interrupt. At first you may sit down to a meal and notice how rushed you feel, how you're barely chewing before you put the next bite into your mouth and how you almost feel unable to control this momentum or do anything about it.

Fast food that's faster than fast

If you're in a hurry, don't have time to prepare a meal and your first inclination to is to 'grab and go' at a fast-food joint, consider an alternative fast food: fruits and vegetables. Fresh fruits make the ultimate fast food:

What's faster than peeling a banana and eating it?

How about washing an apple and biting into it?

What about washing a bowl of grapes?

How about picking up a salad or a wrap?

Or how about making a large smoothie in the morning in under five minutes and taking it with you to sustain yourself throughout the day?

Fast food doesn't have to equal unhealthy food. Create new perceptions around 'convenience' and develop habitual patterns that support your health instead of hindering it.

Mindful awareness is a very positive step in the right direction and gives you the impetus for change. Even if you're not yet ready to adopt new habits, being aware is still better than being unaware and is what precedes your ability to make new choices.

What eating too fast does to your waistline

Eating very quickly has become part of the modern world. These eating habits are established at a young age, with the average school child eating lunch in only seven to ten minutes.

Eating too quickly leads to overeating and lack of satisfaction from your food. Studies by the US Department of Agriculture (USDA) show that on average, people who eat faster have an increased chance of being overweight. This finding is similar to what researchers at Osaka University in Japan discovered through studying the eating habits of 3,000 people. They found that men who ate quickly were 84 percent more likely to be overweight than slower eaters, and women were twice as likely to be overweight as their slower counterparts. These results could be for two primary reasons:

- ✔ When you eat too fast, your body doesn't have sufficient time to signal to your brain that you've had enough. It takes about 20 minutes for the brain to register fullness cues. But oftentimes, calorie-dense meals are gobbled up in a matter of minutes.

- ✔ When you eat in a rush you're activating the part of your nervous system that promotes the release of the stress hormones adrenaline and cortisol. When this happens, blood flow to your stomach decreases, which can impair digestion.

These reasons make slowing down an important skill to nurture and develop.

What slowing down does for your life

In cultures all over the world, people have traditionally honored the process and act of eating. Inherent in this reverence for food is the natural, slow and steady pace that allows you the time to enjoy it.

Within this era of fast food an opposing force has emerged. Known as the Slow Food movement, it originated from Italian culture rooted in traditional ways of living. This movement embodies a *joie de vivre*, a love for life and for all the enjoyable acts sustaining life, such as a love and respect for food and the joys of eating it.

Slow food is more than just about food; it's about embracing a lifestyle that recognizes the great impact our food choices have on our social, economic and environmental systems. This lifestyle is rooted in a greater awareness of the interconnection of all living beings. Living this lifestyle shifts you from 'doing' mode to simply 'being', and enjoying food as a part of a healthy, happy way of life.

Eating calmly and slowly with focused attention is a way that you can cultivate a positive relationship with food. You may start to notice how the flavors of food taste in your mouth as you chew more thoroughly. You may notice more subtleties in what you're eating, like underlying flavors and seasonings. Slowing down allows you to tune in to what your body wants, such as noticing what foods are in season, where they come from and what's fresh and ripe to eat. You allow the time and space for food to enrich your life, playing a meaningful role in your self-care and nourishment.

Tips to mindfully slow down your meals

You can practice slowing down your meals in many ways. Try out all of the suggestions below at least once and keep the practices that most resonate for you. Circle your top three favorite practices to remind yourself to adopt them into your mindful eating routine.

Pay special attention to slowing down and taking your time to eat when you're very hungry (a 1 or 2 on the hunger-fullness scale described earlier in this chapter). When you let yourself get extremely hungry, by mindlessly skipping meals or not paying attention to your hunger signals, you can set yourself up for a potential overeating episode or binge.

✔ **Try to only eat sitting down, at a table if possible:** Even if you're just having a snack, take the extra moment to make it more special by sitting down with your food. Avoid eating in front of the fridge, picking at food while standing at the counter, eating while driving and eating while walking.

✔ **Pause before you eat:** The simple act of pausing before you eat sets the pace for the rest of your meal. Flip to Chapter 11 for more suggestions regarding the power of pausing before you eat.

✔ **Give thanks or say a food blessing:** As outlined previously in this chapter, giving thanks is also a tool for slowing down by pausing before you eat.

✔ **Take time to explore the smells and aroma of your food:** Imagine that you can't eat the food in front of you, only smell it. Do you think you'd take more time to really enjoy all the pleasurable aromas? To describe the smell? Chapter 9 gives an in-depth look at exploring your sense of smell around food.

✔ **Take three deep breaths periodically throughout your meal:** Think about how you typically breathe while you eat. Most people are hard-pressed to give an answer because it's not something they pay attention to. If you don't know, take the opportunity to become more mindful of your breath at your next meal.

✔ **Put your fork or utensil down between bites:** This practice is easy to do, but the key is reminding yourself to do it. What can you set as a reminder to put down your fork? Trying cutting out any shape from a colored piece of paper and placing it next to your plate or bowl as a visual reminder to place your fork down next to it between bites.

✔ **Do you love to masticate?** *Masticate* is a fancy way of saying, 'chew your food'! In the early years of the twentieth century, chewing your food at length became somewhat of a fad diet, popularized by Horace Fletcher, who gave public talks about how much weight he'd lost simply from chewing his food carefully. He coined the term *Fletcherize,* advocating thoroughly chewing your food at least 32 times before swallowing – to be exact!

✔ **Eat with your non-dominant hand:** If you're right-handed try eating with your left hand and vice versa.

✔ **Eat with chopsticks:** This is sure to slow down any newbie to chopsticks. After you become well acquainted with the art of chopsticks, try switching to your non-dominant hand.

✔ **Eat with your hands:** You may want to ditch the eating utensils altogether and simply eat with your hands for a more slow and sensual experience.

✔ **Take a break halfway through your meal:** Who says you have to eat a whole meal all in one shot? By slowing down and pausing halfway through, you allow your body time to process the food in order to signal your brain that you've had enough. You also have a perfect opportunity to use the hunger-fullness scale and check in with how full you are.

✔ **Slower than the slowest:** If you're eating with other people, try to sit back a bit and observe how fast everyone is eating. Try to eat as slowly as, or slower than, the slowest eater. Check out Chapter 11 for more on mindful eating in social situations.

Chapter 9

The Many Ways to Practice Mindful Eating

In This Chapter

▶ Introducing a core mindful eating practice

▶ Experiencing the taste of the last bite of your life

▶ Finding out how to eat mindfully with all of your senses

*I*n this chapter I describe some formal mindful eating practices. Think of these eating exercises as mindfulness meditations if you like – practices in cultivating mindful awareness. I start by exploring a more traditional mindful eating exercise to give you a solid foundation upon which you can build.

Discovering how to consistently keep your attention on what you're experiencing while you eat is one of the primary ways that you strengthen the habit of mindful eating. In this chapter I explore a range of *sensational* eating experiences, allowing you to fine-tune your awareness skills.

Building Your Foundation: A Traditional Mindful Eating Practice

For this introductory mindful eating practice you need one small bite of food. I recommend something like a single raisin, a grape or a cherry. You can also take a single bite from a larger piece of fruit like an apple, a pear or a peach. If using a larger fruit, simply cut off a bite-sized piece before proceeding. Fruit is not only tasty and juicy, but also makes for a pleasurable eating experience. It also encourages you to recognize the delicious sweetness of whole fruit, a healthy substitute for refined sweets.

If you decide to use a stone fruit like a cherry or plum for this exercise, be mindful of the pit!

For this practice, try to look at your chosen food from a young child's perspective, from before you adopted the use of words as labels. Drop the storyline or thought process about the food and have a direct experience without any judgment or added labels of 'good' or 'bad'.

Find a nice, quiet location for this practice, alone or with a mindful eating group (see Chapter 17 for more information on starting a mindful eating group). You can invite a friend or loved one to read the instructions to you or have this book with you at the table and guide yourself through this mindful eating exercise. You can also use a smartphone to record yourself reading the instructions and listen to the recording to guide you through the exercise.

1. Wherever you are, get comfortable. Take three deep breaths and center yourself in the present moment.

2. Pick up this fascinating edible in your hand.

3. Feel the weight of it in your hand. Feel the contact it's making with your skin and your fingers. What does it feel like to hold? What does it feel like to rest it in the palm of your hand?

4. Now explore it with your eyes as if you've never seen this captivating, colorful piece of food before. Look at how it rests in the palm of your hand. Notice the color, the shape, any lines or ridges, the smooth or textured skin, the way it reflects light, the contour.

5. Bring it up to your nose and take a deep breath in. Observe your hand moving up to your face. Notice what the food smells like. Take a few more breaths and notice if the aroma changes.

6. Bring it to your mouth and touch it to your lips. What does it feel like against your lips? Does it feel soft? Does it tickle? Notice if you start to salivate.

7. Gently place this intriguing edible in your mouth and notice what it feels like when it touches your tongue. Are you salivating even more now? What does it feel like when the food touches the different parts of your mouth, like the insides of your cheek, the roof of your mouth or your teeth?

Try to pay attention to what you're experiencing without labeling it or judging. Simply be with the experience with openness and acceptance.

8. When you are ready, slowly take a single bite into this marvelous piece of food. Notice if it makes a sound in your mouth. Notice the flavor that gets released into your mouth. What part of your tongue was the most activated or stimulated from this first bite?

9. Observe the different textures and feel any contrast between the inner and outer part of this bite. Does it have a harder outer skin that contrasts with an inner softness?

10. Bite down again on the morsel in your mouth by chewing very slowly, but at this point, don't swallow.

11. Notice the changing sensations of flavors on the various parts of your tongue.

12. Notice how much you're salivating now.

13. Notice the first impulse to swallow without responding by swallowing the food; instead, keep the food in your mouth. When the impulse to swallow returns, swallow the food when you feel ready to.

14. Notice what it feels like to have this piece of food move all the way down your throat. Follow the sensation as far down your throat as possible, until you can no longer feel it.

15. Continue to slowly chew and swallow until your mouth is cleared. Pay attention to the changing taste sensations in your mouth and notice what aftertaste you experience when you've swallowed your last morsel of the bite. Is there a lingering flavor in your mouth?

After you complete this exercise, open up your mindful eating journal and write about what this exercise was like for you. (Check out Chapter 4 on keeping a journal.) What did you discover? What insights did you have? Nothing is right or wrong. Any experience that you have is completely valid. If you felt bored, tired, distracted, or frustrated, these insights are all as valuable to have as feeling excited, inspired or in awe. How does this eating experience contrast to the way you normally eat?

This exercise forms the basic foundation of mindful eating practices. However, you can explore and experiment with any number of variations, and combine this exercise in any way you desire with the following three mindful eating practices.

You can utilize these mindful eating practices in a very meaningful way to open yourself up to profound insights into your relationship with food. This relationship encompasses and truly embodies and reflects your relationship with life itself.

Fueling your life's purpose

The practice in this section is great as a reflective practice after completing the traditional mindful eating exercise previously outlined. Reflect on the particular questions in this practice as much as possible at the beginning of your mindful eating journey as they provide a powerful impetus for transforming your relationship with food and your life.

Continuing on from the basic mindful eating practice or after you've completed a meal or snack:

1. Close your eyes and imagine the last bite of food moving all the way down your throat and esophagus and into your stomach.

2. Although difficult to fully gasp or comprehend intellectually, reflect on the thousands upon thousands of different interactions and chemical processes that are happening with this food in your body right now. Your whole digestive system is working an incredible miracle to assimilate this food and literally integrate it into your body, making it a part of you.

3. Can you tune in to your inner body awareness and feel what it is like to have this food in your body?

4. Focus your awareness on the energy that is being unlocked and released from this food as it assimilates into your body.

5. Food is literally fuel for your body. Without it, you can't wake up every day, spend time with your family or do the things you love. Reflect on how your body uses the energy from this food that you've just eaten to enable you to move, to feel and to think – essentially to sustain your life.

6. Can you feel how special this connection is with your food source?

7. Now ask yourself: 'How am I spending this precious energy in my life? Am I doing something I value with this energy? Something that makes me truly happy? Am I using this food to fuel and support a deeper purpose in my life?'

Allow yourself as much time as you need to sit with these self-reflective questions. I encourage you to open up your mindful eating journal and write whatever you're feeling in this moment. Does this practice shift your relationship with food at all? Can you see what a gift and blessing food is, rather than something you struggle with or try to control?

Total interconnection

Mindful eating can help you become aware of a very fundamental and important reality – the interconnectivity that everything shares. (The sidebar 'Interbeing' discusses total interconnection in more depth.) Food becomes part of a larger spiritual practice and brings deeper meaning into your life when explored within this realm of reality. Mindfulness allows you to honor the food you eat, and thus honor yourself, changing the way you relate to food and the relationship you have with food.

You can use the following mindful eating exercise of total interconnection as a stand-alone practice or as a continuation from the earlier one-bite mindful eating exercise, using whatever bite of whole food you tasted.

Interbeing

The Vietnamese Zen Buddhist monk and author Thich Nhat Hanh is known for coining the term *interbeing*. This term refers to the interconnectedness of all things and is a central concept taught in the Buddhist tradition.

Thich Nhat Hanh frequently uses a flower to explain this concept of interbeing. In your mind's eye, think about a sunflower. When you think about a flower, you tend to see only the flower, but when you look more closely, you can see that this flower is actually made up of the entire universe. It's made up of the rain, which is connected to the clouds and oceans and other large bodies of water. It's made up of soil, which is connected with all the elements that came together over time to make up that soil, including countless years of plants, animals and smaller insects that decomposed in that soil providing nutrients for the earth to become fertile enough to hold space for the manifestation of a beautiful flower. Each of these causes had other causes, and, in turn, these causes had causes, extending out to encompass all the elements in the universe. The flower does not exist alone, in isolation. If you were to take away all of these elements you would no longer have a flower; it would cease to exist.

The same holds true for us as humans, for animals, for our food and everything else in the universe, making this one large, interconnected codependent web that we call life.

1. Look at the food in front of you and imagine and connect to the plant that grew this food. Do you know what it looks like?

2. Imagine yourself traveling back in time to the moment that this plant was a seed. Imagine the previous plant that created this seed, and the plant before that and the plant before that.

3. Consider how this plant's flowers were pollinated. In order for most plants to bear fruits and vegetables, they need to be pollinated by a specific insect. These tiny pollinators, including bees, butterflies, moths and even ants, play a crucial role in providing us with our food supply.

4. Come back to imagining the plant that this food came from and visualize the soil that supported the roots of this plant. Imagine all the elements in the soil that provide nutrients for the plant to grow.

5. Imagine the rain falling and being absorbed by the soil and hydrating the plant through its roots.

6. Picture where that water came from, the cloud that carried the water, and the ocean or large body of water that the cloud came from. Contemplate how that body of water is connected to the rivers, streams, lakes and mountains all over the world.

7. Visualize the sun's heat and energy penetrating the plant and all the chemical reactions that help the plant grow.

8. Now imagine all the people who partook in cultivating this plant and the food it's created. Think of every person who propagated this seed over the many generations; the person who planted this specific seed; the farmer who cultivated it or watered it; the farm worker who picked it; the people who packed, shipped, displayed and sold it.

9. Reflect on the millions of synchronicities that had to align and come together to bring this piece of food to you. This food is the result of countless conditions temporarily coming together and aligning at a precise moment in time. This food in front of you is directly connected to the whole universe.

After you complete this exercise, grab your mindful eating journal and reflect on how this practice may have changed or shifted your perspective on food. Did it allow you to have more gratitude and appreciation for the food? Does it impact the way you look at how you are connected to nature and the food you eat?

Last bite of your life

You know the famous saying that goes something along the lines of, 'You never know how good you have it, until it's gone'? When you've become accustomed to something, you don't fully appreciate it, and if you've never gone without it, you tend to take it for granted. This attitude also most certainly applies to your body. How much do you appreciate *not* having a sore stomach as soon as your stomach hurts? Do you notice how much you take your health for granted when you spend the day sick in bed? Do you notice how grateful you can become for ease of mobility when you hurt a foot?

The same rings true for food and eating. Because people eat multiple times every single day, they tend to forget the inherent magic in each and every bite. They very rarely *fully* taste a single bite of food. They tend to forget and thus disregard the specialness that each bite has to offer us.

The following exercise is a fun mindful eating exercise that you can do on your own, with friends or turn into a game to play with your kids. You can practice 'last bite of your life' with actual food or as a visualization exercise; both are effective.

Imagine that you've just got home from the doctor who has informed you that you are about to lose the functioning of your taste buds. You only have one meal left to taste, enjoy and experience, and then that's it – your ability to taste is gone forever!

With your meal in front of you:

1. Notice how you approach this meal differently.

2. Notice how you take your time to look at the food, including all the colors and textures on the plate.

3. If it's a warm meal, notice if you can witness the delicate wisps of steam rising off the food.

4. Do you notice yourself paying more attention and making more of an effort to be present and fully experience this meal?

5. Take in the smell of this food. Are you taking more time to enjoy the aroma coming from your meal?

6. Notice the movement of your hand picking up your utensils. If you're eating with your hands, feel what that food is like when it touches your fingers.

7. Take your first bite. Are you taking more time to properly chew and extract as much taste out of this bite as possible?

8. Do you notice yourself moving slower than you normally do?

9. Do you notice yourself pausing more between bites?

10. Observe what thoughts are going through your mind. Are you recognizing how lucky you've been to enjoy the pleasure of eating all these years?

What do you notice about this experience? Open your mindful eating journal and grab a pen and describe your experience and what you discovered. Add any thoughts, comments and reflections that you may have about this experience.

Tasting Your Senses

Your senses are very important. Essentially, you experience your reality through your senses. How you experience life can be thought of as how your brain processes and interprets the information that comes through your senses. Just as your senses shape your experience of life, they also shape your relationship with food and eating.

One of the ways you become more mindful is through exploring your senses and finding out how to tune in to them both individually and collectively. Fortunately, eating offers a full sensory experience, engaging each one of your five senses. Therefore eating is the perfect opportunity to be fully engaged with the present moment rather than another occasion for mindlessness. Even if you're busy throughout your day, eating can act as a trigger to remind you to become mindful and aware of the 'now' moments of your life.

Through these mindful eating exercises, you can explore each of your senses and discover how to tune in to and become aware of each one, offering you a full experience of the present moment and a rich experience when eating.

In the following section, we will explore the sights, smells, sounds and tastes of food.

 Mindfulness includes having a non-judgmental attitude about what you're experiencing. When exploring your senses, simply observe and witness whatever you're experiencing without labeling or thinking about it. See if you can simply let go of any thought process or story-line about what it is that you're experiencing and be with the present moment and whatever it's offering you. If you do notice yourself thinking, which inevitably happens, just remind yourself to come back to your senses!

Exploring sight: colors and delight

Your eyes play a very intimate role in your eating behavior. I'm sure that you're familiar with sayings like, 'Your eyes are bigger than your stomach' when you allow your eyes to dictate how much you should eat without consulting the hunger levels of your stomach. Your eating is constantly based on visual cues, including how food looks, how much food you have left on your plate, how much food is out on the table, how much variety of food you perceive around you, as well as how much food you see other people eating.

Think about the last time you took more food than you were actually hungry for. When you noticed yourself starting to get full, what did you decide to do? Reflect on how often you tend to continue to eat past fullness simply because the food *looks* so good or because you'd rather see an empty plate than a plate with food left on it.

Taking a moment before you eat to really drink in your meal with your eyes is an excellent way to become grounded in the present moment. At your next meal, before you eat, take a moment to explore your food with your eyes. Notice the colors, the reflecting light, the contour, shapes and ridges of your food. Notice what the texture looks like. Pay attention to whether looking at this food is making you desire the food more. Notice if you start to salivate just by looking at the food. On a scale of 1 to 10, with 10 being the most, how appealing does this food look to you? What about it is appealing or less appealing to you?

When your eyes are bigger than your stomach

Repeated studies conducted by Cornell University Food and Brand Lab, led by founder Brian Wansink, have shown that people who eat off of bigger plates, as well as out of bigger packages and serving containers, eat more food than they do from comparatively smaller dishes. This phenomenon is so powerful that even when people are educated about this bias, they still tend to eat more! In fact, even when the food doesn't taste pleasant, if they're eating out of a larger container, they habitually eat more. This problem is growing (no pun intended) because of the increased portion sizes served in restaurants, as well as the increase in size of the average American plate by over three inches in diameter in only the past few decades.

If you notice yourself constantly overeating, downsize to a smaller plate or bowl. Eat with a smaller spoon or fork. Keep your larger plates and bowls for when you're eating low-calorie, nutrient-dense water- and fiber-rich foods like fruits and vegetables to encourage yourself to eat more of those foods.

Are your eyes deceiving you?

Considering how much you can 'eat with your eyes', it's not surprising to discover that studies conducted to explore the relationship of the eyes with food consumption reveal that obese subjects ate almost 25 percent less food when blindfolded! The blindfold can make for a very interesting (and perhaps messy) mindful eating exercise, although one that I highly recommend!

By simply closing your eyes, you allow your awareness to shift inward. Much of the time, the feedback that you receive from your eyes encourages you to keep eating. Closing your eyes can help you turn your attention away from the visual cues of eating, which are often unrelated to hunger, and tune in to your hunger and fullness levels, enabling you to develop a stronger connection with your inner body awareness. (Chapter 8 covers checking you hunger and fullness levels.)

Your eyes can also play tricks on you and influence how you experience a meal based on how you perceive it. In one experiment, French researchers fooled even the so-called experts. They colored a white wine with an odorless red dye and invited the wine connoisseurs to describe its taste. Not surprisingly, they described it using characteristic red wine descriptors rather than the more appropriate white wine descriptors. This type of experiment has been done in many different ways to fool people's perceptions of the taste of food, including a vanilla yogurt dyed pink to influence the perception of a strawberry flavor. This effect is one of the reasons why food dyes are so highly used in the processed-food industry; people are encouraged to think a food tastes how it is supposed to, based on the color, not the flavor.

One way you can discover how much your eyes influence your eating behavior is by *not* using them when eating a meal.

The following mindful eating exercise is a lot of fun with a group of people and is definitely one to try alone or with your family, friends or mindful eating group.

Prepare a meal and a blindfold for each person participating. Allow everyone to prepare their own plates without their blindfold. Then when everyone is sitting, invite everyone to cover their eyes with the blindfolds. Ask everyone to check in with how hungry they are (flip to Chapter 8 for how to tune in to hunger and fullness levels) and proceed to eat slowly. The participants should stop when they're full. After everyone is finished, open up a discussion by asking everyone to notice how much food is still on their plates and what they noticed that was different from eating without a blindfold.

Visually pleasurable

A lot of the satisfaction that you receive from food comes from the way it looks and is presented. Chefs from all over the world spend years of their lives exploring and pushing the limits of food presentation as an art form. The way food is displayed and how appealing it looks can and does influence not only your eating behavior, but also how much you think you enjoy a food.

Imagine yourself at a restaurant; you're relatively full from dinner when the dessert cart rolls around. On one plate sits a decadent piece of chocolate cake, presented in a beautiful manner, while on another plate sits the same cake, but mashed up into a big dark blob of gooiness. Which one do you think you'd prefer? If you only saw the second plate and didn't know it was mashed-up chocolate cake, would you find it appetizing? Why do you think that is?

We constantly use our eyes as reinforcement to help us determine what we're about to eat and how much pleasure we think we're going to derive from it.

No matter what it is you're eating, make an effort to arrange your food in a nice way on an attractive serving dish. Whether you're eating a snack, take out or leftovers, make the little extra effort to beautify your meal. If you're pouring yourself a glass of water or juice, why not use a nice glass, or even a wine glass for that matter? Put down a nice table cloth or place mat. Can you beautify your surroundings by also lighting a candle or placing a flower arrangement on the table?

Watching out for food ads

The sight of food is a very powerful trigger for some people. Marketers know this all too well and use images of food to evoke powerful emotions and trigger us to eat.

Food advertisements can lure almost anyone to eat when they're not hungry. Studies show that people who watch more commercial television eat more junk food and snack more following exposure to food advertisements – and not even necessarily on the food that was shown in the commercial. These results don't bode well for today's youth. (Take a look at the nearby sidebar 'Are food ads influencing childhood obesity?' for more.) Thankfully, mindful eating can really help in these types of situations.

Start to notice what images of foods trigger you to want to eat. Do you notice yourself seeking out food after you've watched TV, read recipes online or scanned through a magazine?

Are food ads influencing childhood obesity?

According to a study conducted by the Kaiser Family Foundation, every year the average American child watches between 30 and 50 hours of food commercials on TV – 90 percent of which are for junk food, and none of which are for fruits and vegetables. Children are bombarded with ads to eat junk food and consume sugary drinks.

More and more studies are linking these ads to the many weight issues our youth now face as obesity rates amongst children are at an all-time high and are rising at an alarming rate.

According to the Center for Disease Control (CDC), childhood obesity has more than doubled in children and quadrupled in adolescents in the past 30 years, and in 2012, more than one third of children and adolescents in the US were overweight or obese. This puts children at risk for a wide range of health complications and diseases, including cardiovascular disease, type 2 diabetes and osteoarthritis, not to mention potential social and psychological problems and potential low self-esteem.

Exploring smell: What's cooking?

Have you ever experienced walking into a movie theater and all of a sudden – wham – the smell of popcorn fills your nose and immediately provokes your knee-jerk 'I want that now' reaction?

Nothing thrusts you into the present moment like a really intense smell – whether pleasant or unpleasant. Your sense of smell is another sensory doorway into mindful awareness that you can practice concentrating on to help become more mindful of your relationship with food and eating.

Smelling the taste of food

Have you ever noticed that when you're sick, food doesn't quite taste the same? When you're congested, your nasal passageway can become blocked, which actually influences how you taste your food because the way that you taste food and its flavor is actually in large part a result of your sense of smell. Although your senses of smell and taste have separate receptor organs, they are nonetheless highly influenced by each other.

When you first encounter food, you breathe in its aroma up through the nose and then into the mouth, which allows you to anticipate its flavor and to determine if this is going to be an enjoyable experience or not, or if this is a food that should be avoided. Since the beginning of time, people and many animals alike have used their sense of smell as an instinctive survival-based mechanism to protect against rotten, spoiled or poisonous food. (Check out the sidebar 'Durian fruit: A rotten delicacy?' for an exception to the rule – a highly nutritious but rotten-smelling food!)

Part of the reason that you perceive aroma and smell as flavor is because when you eat foods, the airborne odor molecules, called *odorants*, that the food releases travel up past the nasal passage into a part of the brain called the *olfactory bulb* that interprets it as flavor. So, for example, if a sweet odor is added to a particular food, it acts to increase the *perception* of sweet taste.

Durian fruit: A rotten delicacy?

If you've ever been to a tropical area like Thailand or Hawaii you may have come across a very intriguing fruit called durian.

Durian offers a complexity of both aroma and flavor and elicits a wide spectrum of responses. Most people liken its smell to dirty socks or rotten sewage, and you can get kicked off buses or out of hotels or bars for carrying one with you. On the other end of the spectrum, despite the rotten smell, some people go crazy for this fruit, considering it a delicacy and paying a hefty price for a single fruit. Many people say that if you can get past the smell and actually taste it, you may rethink your opinion of durian.

Although the smell does indeed influence the taste of the durian, it makes for a unique eating experience that people tend to love or hate, but rarely forget!

Imagine that the only way you can experience nourishment from food is through smelling it.

- ✔ With your food in front of you, take your time to try to smell and explore the full range of aromas being released from the food.

- ✔ Notice the dynamic play of smells between ingredients.

- ✔ Notice if the aroma shifts and changes as you continue to smell your food.

- ✔ Does smelling your food influence your hunger level?

- ✔ If you have a meal in front of you, try to name the different ingredients simply through smelling your food.

- ✔ Try to describe what this food smells like in as much detail as possible, out loud to others, to yourself or in your mindful eating journal.

- ✔ Notice if this smell is triggering any pleasant or unpleasant emotions in you.

- ✔ Notice if this smell is triggering any pleasant or unpleasant memories.

- ✔ What does this smell remind you of?

- ✔ Do you consider this smell to be pleasant, unpleasant or neutral?

Did you know that humans can detect more than 10,000 different aromas? Some of the aromas that you may detect in food include: fresh, moldy, fruity, spoiled, pungent, artificial, cooked, canned, green or earthy, woody, floral, seedy, nutty, caramelized, sulfurous, garlic, alcoholic and acidic, just to name a few. Is this shifting your perspective as to the incredibly wide range of smells that you can detect in your food? Get creative and start to notice what aromas you smell in your food.

In today's marketing-oriented food environment, food companies quite commonly intentionally implant artificial aromas right into their food packaging to try to influence a more positive eating experience and in turn encourage consumers to eat more than they actually need to. Now that you're more aware of how smell influences your eating experience, pay special attention to how manufactured pleasant food smells may be encouraging you to eat more than you're actually hungry for.

The next time you notice a craving being stimulated or activated through a food's smell, try blocking your nose and tasting the food again and notice how the eating experience changes for you. If it's a packaged food you're eating, try putting a smaller portion on a nice plate and remove the package and all the smells it emanates from the eating experience. Do you notice a difference in how you perceive the flavor and taste of the food?

Smells like comfort

Part of the reason that smell is so strongly linked to your emotions is because the olfactory bulb previously mentioned is embedded within the part of the brain where emotions are stored, making your sense of a smell a powerful influencer in terms of what, when and how much you choose to eat.

There's nothing like walking into a home that's saturated in the smells of delicious home cooking. Whether it's a pot of soup on the stove, a roasting turkey or fresh-baked bread in the oven, these smells have the strength to evoke powerful memories in us, often special ones from childhood.

Make a list of the smells of particular foods that evoke the most emotional reaction in you, whether pleasant or unpleasant. What memories do these smells trigger in you? How does it make you feel to smell them? Does it encourage you to go on automatic pilot and mindlessly eat that particular food? Does it trigger you to eat in unhealthy ways? Do these smells trigger you to overeat? Do the smells of these particular foods make you feel loved, lonely, sad, happy or angry? Explore these mindful eating questions in your journal along with any other thoughts that may be helpful for self-reflection.

Exploring sound: Music to your mouth

Many traditions use a bell or a gong in meditation practice, not only to initiate or end a meditation session, but also to serve as a reminder to be present. Sounds can instantly bring your awareness into the present moment. Mindfulness meditations that use sound as a centralized focus can help remind you to listen to the world around you as a way to be present here rather than lost in thought.

It's amazing how easily you can learn to tune sounds out, especially if you live in a city with constant background noise. But you can use any sound as a way to ground yourself in the present moment, as long as you shift your attention towards it. Sometimes you don't even have to try. You can be going about automatically, and then all of a sudden an unexpected or loud noise happens, or you hear a unique bird song or a really funny laugh. In the instant that the sound catches your attention, you experience mindful awareness of the present moment. Reaching and maintaining those moments of pure awareness for as long as possible is the essence of mindfulness.

Put down your book and take one minute to listen to the sounds around you. Focus your attention on sounds happening farther away, perhaps outside your house. Now shift your attention towards sounds happening closer, maybe in your house or in your room. What do you hear?

You may experience an infinite number of sounds that relate to food, whether in food preparation, during a meal or after a meal while cleaning up. In the same way that a meditation bell can help remind meditators to become present, you can use food-related sounds to help remind you to become aware of what you're doing in the present moment. Eating, and all the acts surrounding eating, therefore can become an active meditation, a part of your everyday life.

At your next meal, pay extra attention to all of the sounds associated with eating. You may notice sounds during:

- **Cooking and meal preparation:** Vegetables frying in a pan, a blender mixing a smoothie, spoons clanging against a bowl as you toss a salad, a knife hitting the cutting board as you chop up vegetables, a kettle whistling or popcorn popping.

- **Eating:** all the different sounds of chewing food, biting into a crunchy apple or a crispy chip, slurping a soup or a cup of tea, swallowing, your knife and fork tapping against your plate or a spoon against a bowl.

- **Cleaning up:** running water, washing dishes, scraping food off a plate or loading the dishwasher.

Paying special attention to the sounds that you notice while you're actually eating is a wonderful technique to help focus your awareness on the experience of eating.

In your mindful eating journal, make a list of five distinct sounds you noticed during your last meal. Also note if you were distracted by other sounds that were unrelated to your meal that made it difficult for you to be present with your food.

Being distracted by conversation and noise around you is quite common. The more you practice these mindful eating exercises, the more you start to become aware of these distractions and discover how to redirect your focus towards your food and eating experience. Look at Chapter 8 for more on removing distractions and Chapter 11 on how to eat mindfully in social situations.

Start to pay attention to how certain sounds may trigger food cravings. If you hear someone opening up a bag of chips (crisps), does this trigger something in you to want to reach for a bag of chips as well? Starting to pay attention to all of your food triggers helps you to notice what may be triggering you to mindlessly eat and therefore make better, more informed food-related choices. Check out Chapter 3 for more about food triggers.

Exploring taste: A burst of juicy joy

Finally, taste – the reason why you love to eat. Your sense of taste has a strong connection to the pleasure centers in your brain and strongly influences not only how much you enjoy food, but also how much you eat – whether you're full or not.

Aside from providing pleasure, taste also protects you from eating spoiled or rotten foods, so preventing you from getting sick. Think of your eyes and nose as your first line of protective defense and taste as your second line of defense against harmful substances.

Tasting taste

Taste is detected by receptor cells called taste buds that are located primarily on the tongue. Your taste buds have chemical receptors that detect specific molecules in food, allowing you to classify taste sensations into five primary categories:

- ✔ **Sweet:** signals the presence of sugars; found in fruits, milk, grains and root vegetables.

- ✔ **Salty:** signals sodium ions in the food; found in table salt, soy sauce, salted meats and fish and the majority of packaged foods.

- ✔ **Sour:** indicates acidity; naturally found in sour foods like lemons, limes, grapefruit, green apples, tamarind and passion fruit.

- ✔ **Bitter:** is the most sensitive of the tastes and may be described as sharp or pungent; found in dark, leafy vegetables, cacao and coffee.

- ✔ **Umami:** is the most recent addition to the descriptive taste categories and is described as savory. Umami is found in cheese, soy sauce, tomatoes, grains, beans and foods containing monosodium glutamate (MSG), which was developed as a food additive in the early 1900s.

 Start to train your palate to distinguish between the five different tastes. When you're eating, see if you can detect which of the five primary tastes are present in your food. See if you can notice the different parts of your tongue that are activated by the different tastes. Do you taste sweetness on a different part of your tongue than you do salty or bitter flavors?

Is it the flavor you're tasting?

Although often thought of as the same thing, taste and flavor are different and have their own unique qualities. Most of the time when you're talking about taste, what you're actually describing is flavor. Describing flavor is less straightforward than taste and is open to much more descriptive interpretation.

Flavor is a combination of three primary senses that include:

- **Taste:** the five basic taste categories. Experts estimate that taste accounts for roughly 5 to 20 percent of perceived flavor.

- **Smell:** the aroma from smelling food and from actually eating food plays a dominant role in flavor. Some experts say that aroma can account for anywhere from 50 to 90 percent of perceived flavor.

- **Touch:** the way that we experience mouthfeel while eating. Mouthfeel provide us with tactile information and is comprised of several factors including:

    a. Texture: crunchy, smooth, solid, liquid, creamy, crumbly, dry, grainy, gummy, cohesive, hard, soft, rough, slippery, moist, heavy, dense and so on.

    b. Temperature: hot, warm or cold.

    c. Level of irritation: spicy or cooling.

    d. Astringency: causes a dry and puckering mouthfeel from tannins found in certain fruits, wines and teas.

Mouthfeel is estimated to account for roughly 5 to 20 percent of perceived flavor.

Think of each bite you take as a taste-testing experiment. Dive deep into exploring the flavor of food with curiosity, using your senses as your guide. The more you start to pay attention to all the different qualities of flavor, the more you start to notice the many subtleties and the myriad different combinations that can come together to offer you a uniquely flavorful experience.

First bite awareness

Consistently returning your attention to what you're tasting in your mouth is one of the foundations of mindful eating. Becoming distracted is all too easy, and eating without actually experiencing eating leaves you feeling dissatisfied, discontent and wanting more.

At your next meal or snack, try this 'first bite awareness' exercise: Notice how the first bite tastes and notice how satisfying (or unsatisfying) it is. Notice if, when you're mind wanders, your satisfaction and enjoyment is reduced. Notice if the second bite tastes as good as the first. Notice if the third bite tastes as good as the first or second. At what point do your taste satisfaction, pleasure and enjoyment start to decline? Grab your mindful eating journal and jot down any thoughts about what this exercise taught you.

Part IV
Mindful Eating, Mindful Life

Top five ways to adopt mindful eating into your everyday life

- ✔ **Adopt mindful eating in your home and family environment:** practicing mindful eating with your family, especially children, helps encourage everyone to eat with more awareness and sets a good example for building a healthy and balanced relationship with food.

- ✔ **Discover how to navigate mindful eating in social outings that revolve around food:** we all know that most social situations these days include food. These situations also offer lots in the way of distractions, making it more challenging to be present with the act of eating.

- ✔ **Use mindful eating to work with food cravings:** for many people, food cravings are no laughing matter and can have the power to cause pain and hardship in one's life. Mindful eating is a very helpful tool to deal with cravings when they arise.

- ✔ **Use mindfulness to help you overcome setbacks:** Chapter 12 contains some great tools to help you get back on track if your eating habits take a turn in a direction that you're not so thrilled about.

- ✔ **Apply mindful eating to help reverse emotional eating habits:** emotions are a part of the human experience and often food and eating can become enmeshed in a wide range of emotional experiences.

Get information on starting a mindful eating group to share your experiences and get support from others at www.dummies.com/extras/mindfuleating.

In this part . . .

- Find out how to apply mindful eating within the context of your everyday life.

- Explore mindful eating with your family and children.

- Discover how to navigate social situations that revolve around food more mindfully.

- Apply mindfulness during challenging social situations, such as eating in restaurants, during the holidays and whilst travelling.

- Find time for mindful eating within a busy schedule.

- Mindfully work with food cravings.

- Mindfully explore emotional hunger and your emotional triggers to eat.

Chapter 10

Mindful Eating for Families

● ●

In This Chapter

▶ Cultivating a positive mindful eating environment at home

▶ Enjoying mindful mealtimes with your family

▶ Exploring mindful eating with your kids

● ●

Sharing meals as a family can be a very special time for both children and parents. Parents get an opportunity to engage with their kids and be present for what's happening in their lives. Children feel that they have their parents' attention and are being listened to. Mealtimes become a special time of nourishment and connection where fond memories are created. The significance of this simple act has made sharing family meals a tradition in cultures all over the world for many generations past.

In today's increasingly fast-paced culture, that tradition is slowly being lost as family-shared meals are becoming less and less frequent. These days, both parents in the household quite commonly work full-time jobs. Couple this with extended working hours and long commutes, and understandably many parents are often too tired to prepare meals at the end of the day or help children prepare their lunches. As children become teenagers, their lives also naturally become increasingly busier with sports, after school activities and spending more time with friends.

Cultivating a Mindful Eating Environment at Home

When family meals are shared, enjoying them together in a mindful way is very important. The environment that surrounds meals can strongly influence a child's long-term relationship with food. Often times, when family meals are shared, they revolve around television, the Internet, cell phones (mobiles), arguments or disagreements and other constant distractions. When meals are dominated by distractions everyone misses the special level of nourishment and connection that family meals can inherently provide. Practicing mindful eating with the family instills positive lifelong habits around eating and sets everyone up to have a healthy relationship with food.

Benefiting from shared meals

Reconnecting to the tradition of shared family meals has many positive benefits for the whole family. Research indicates that sharing family meals is an essential component of a healthy lifestyle. When families eat together, everyone tends to eat healthier – more fruits and vegetables and less consumption of soda and fried foods. Children are also less likely to be depressed and overweight and less likely to skip out on breakfast.

At some point you need to ask yourself what the benefits are of a busy and hectic lifestyle compared to what you stand to lose by not establishing a routine family connection over shared meals.

Close your eyes and think back to when you were a child. Did you share meals with your family? What do you remember about mealtimes? Was eating as a family generally pleasant or unpleasant? How do you think your family shaped your relationship with food?

Creating an atmosphere for mindful eating

Create a mood that is set around eating, food preparation and mealtime. This atmosphere is attitude-related and can set the tone for an enjoyable eating experience.

A fisherman's tale

Once upon a time, an American tourist was traveling in a small town on the Mexican coast. He notices a small boat with a fisherman pull up to the dock with several nice-sized fish. The tourist compliments the fisherman and asks him how long it took him to catch those fish.

'Not very long,' the fisherman replies.

'Why not stay out longer and catch more fish to make more money?' the tourist asks him.

'Because I have enough to meet my family's needs.'

The tourist thinks about this for a moment and then asks the fisherman: 'What do you do with all your spare time?'

The fisherman smiles and explains that he spends time with his children, playing music, resting and sharing family meals together. He is proud to say he has a full and rewarding life with his family.

The tourist explains that he's a banker, and he can help the fisherman find more happiness for himself and his family. The banker explains that the fisherman can take out a loan, work longer hours catching more fish and use the proceeds and the loan to buy a bigger boat. Eventually, the fisherman will have enough to buy a whole fleet of boats and have employees working for him. He would have to move or commute to a bigger city, where he could more effectively manage his growing business and have access to his customers.

The fisherman ponders this for a moment, then asks: 'How long will this take?' To which the tourist replies, 'Only 20 to 25 years. Then you can eventually retire and sell your business to a bigger company for a lot of money.'

'And then what?' the fisherman asks with a puzzled look on his face.

'Then you can have time to spend with your children, play music, rest and share meals with your family.'

This parable points towards what so many of us do in our culture; sacrifice a simple lifestyle in order to work hard to earn the privilege of enjoying the same simple pleasures in life.

Try to foster a mindful eating environment at home that is:

✔ **Positive:** create an uplifting, inspiring environment that is focused on positive reinforcement.

✔ **Empowering:** encourage children to tune in with themselves and make food-related decisions that they feel are best for them.

✔ **Supportive:** support the food-related decisions that children make that are health-focused.

✔ **Informative:** educate your children about making healthy food choices.

✔ **Mindful:** encourage children to engage all of their senses and pay attention to the act of eating.

✔ **Accepting:** Listen to children express whatever they need to express without judgment.

✔ **Calm:** create a peaceful eating environment. Creating time for families to eat together without everyone feeling rushed is important.

✔ **Loving:** be gentle, kind and loving with your communication around meal times.

Mixing food with emotionally intense situations is best avoided at the dinner table. If something needs to be addressed, make an agreement to finish the meal and discuss it afterwards or put the meal on hold until the discussion is over so that you and your family can pay mindful attention to your food and try to avoid mixing food with negative emotions.

Try to eat at least one meal per day with the whole family or with as many family members present as possible. If eating weekday meals together is becoming less realistic, allocate Sunday afternoon and evenings as family dinnertime.

Removing distractions

To add to a positive eating atmosphere, add to the ambiance by removing distractions like television, games, loud music and electronic devices. With children as young as six years old starting to carry cell phones, setting a 'no cell phones' policy at the dinner table is becoming increasingly appropriate. Mindful mealtimes are for directing attention toward the experience of eating.

Sometimes nice music playing in the background can really add to an enjoyable mealtime experience. Make sure that everyone present is okay with soft background music and choose music that is uplifting, not too distracting and not too loud so that people don't have to talk loudly to be heard.

The power of giving thanks

Establishing mindful rituals into your family's eating routine is a powerful way to set a positive tone for the rest of the meal and fosters a strong foundation of mindfulness in the home environment. Raising children to bless their food before they eat helps to cultivate an attitude of gratitude, appreciation for the food and for the people gathered to share it. Everyone is allowed to slow down, pause and take a deep breath before eating. Chapter 8 contains more about giving thanks before meals.

Make a commitment to set a good example for your family by giving thanks for your food before you eat. You can make giving thanks for food fun for children in many ways.

For instance, have a mealtime blessing song that you sing with your children. Rhymes and songs are easier for children to remember. It doesn't have to be long; it can be short and sweet and right to the point!

> *Thank you for the world so sweet,*
>
> *Thank you for the food we eat,*
>
> *Thank you, thank you, thank you,*
>
> *Bon appétit,*
>
> *Now we may eat!*

> *Bless this food and the earth that grew it,*
>
> *Thank you Mother Earth for sustaining me.*
>
> *As we sit in awe of abundance,*
>
> *We can all eat in harmony.*

You can ask for a single volunteer to say the blessing or go around the circle and give everyone an opportunity to say one thing that they're grateful for. This habit encourages children to participate and offers them an opportunity to practice expressing gratitude for the food.

Giving thanks as a family before meals instills thoughtfulness and contemplation of the greater interconnection we all share to each other, to this earth and with our food. You can teach children about this interconnection through mealtime blessings. Check out Chapter 8 for suggestions on the different ways to give thanks before meals.

Moment of silence

Another wonderful practice that supports and fosters an atmosphere for mindful eating is the power of silence. As a family, explore a moment of silence after you say a blessing or give thanks and encourage everyone to feast with their eyes on the food and notice all the wonderful smells coming from the table. You may also want to explore taking a moment of silence while you start eating, or both!

At your next meal, invite your family to eat the first two minutes of the meal in silence. People can then really tune in to and connect with their food. You may notice people reveling in the sensory pleasure of their food with *mmmmm*s and *ahhhhhh*s! After the two minutes is up, ring a bell or tap your glass lightly with a fork and invite people to share their experiences of this silent eating exercise.

Focus on the food

Another practice to instill at your shared family meals is to direct the focus of attention on the food. This practice is a nice follow-up to taking a moment of silence where you can then focus the conversation around the food or enjoy fun mindful eating games with your kids.

Explore these questions with your children:

- ✔ Describe the smell of your food before you taste it.
- ✔ Try to name the spice or seasoning in this dish.
- ✔ Name the vegetables you see on your plate.
- ✔ What's your favorite part of this meal?
- ✔ What's your least favorite part of this meal?
- ✔ Can you describe the texture of a bite?
- ✔ What textures do you like the best?

You can also focus on more thought-provoking conversation, depending on the age of your children.

- ✔ How far has this food travelled to reach this table?
- ✔ How many people do you think were involved to allow this food to reach the table?
- ✔ What natural elements went into helping this food grow?

You can also explore a wide range of health- and food-related topics, more geared towards older children. Often these more thought-provoking questions are best discussed after the meal is finished, while everyone is still sitting at the table.

- ✔ What does a healthy dietary lifestyle include?
- ✔ What are the benefits of organic foods over conventionally grown foods?
- ✔ What are genetically modified organisms (GMOs) and what, if any, are the associated health and environmental risks?
- ✔ What does eating sustainably involve?
- ✔ Is it ethical to eat animals?

Mindful Eating with Kids

Babies and young children are expert mindful eaters. Infants are especially good at knowing when they're hungry and when they've had enough, as well as what they like and dislike based on their bodies' needs. You were born with a strong intuitive connection to your body that guided you to make food-related choices. Even before you could speak, you communicated to others when you were hungry by crying and when you had had enough by naturally pulling away.

As you get older, your thinking mind often overrides your feeling body as you become inundated with diet and nutrition-related information. This information is often highly contradictory, leaving you very confused about what and how much to eat. As a result your food-related belief system gets in the way of a once healthy relationship with your body and with food.

Parents have a strong influence on their children's attitudes towards food and eating. Young children are very impressionable, and that's why setting a good example is very important so that children can develop and strengthen their mindful eating habits before they start learning mindless eating habits from us adults!

In addition to what you can teach children about mindful eating, remember that adults have much to learn from their children as well! The mindful eating environment at home then becomes a mutually supportive and beneficial relationship that the whole family can participate in and benefit from.

Resigning from the 'clean your plate' fan club

Are you a member of the 'clean your plate' fan club? Do you have a hard time leaving food on your plate, despite being full? Where do you think this behavior was developed? Most people learned this mindless eating habit at home as their parents routinely reminded them to 'Finish what's on your plate!' Parents often use guilt-inducing reminders like:

- ✔ Eat your food! There are children starving in Africa.

- ✔ Throwing away food is wasteful, and we don't have money to waste.

- ✔ Finish your plate; that food was expensive, and I worked hard to buy that for you.

- ✔ We never had the luxury of eating like this when we were kids. You're lucky to have meals like this.

- ✔ Finish your plate sweetie. I worked so hard to make that food just for you. Don't you want to eat my food? Don't you like it?

Making remarks like this can turn children into guilty eaters, setting them up for a lifelong unhealthy or disordered relationship with food. This 'clean your plate' mentality teaches children to ignore their inherent body wisdom and to proceed to eat until they reach the external visual cue of an empty plate.

Think back to when you were a kid. Did your parents encourage you to clean your plate? How do you think these messages affected your long-term relationship with food? If you're a parent or work with children, notice in what ways you may be encouraging the same mentality. What routine lines do you use with your children to encourage them to clean their plates? Perhaps initiate an open dialogue with your children and ask them how it makes them feel when you say things like that.

Listening to children when they communicate that they've had enough without pressuring them to keep eating past fullness is important. A great place to start is to teach children the hunger-fullness scale presented in Chapter 8. Teaching kids this technique in a fun and playful way encourages them to get in touch with their inner body awareness around hunger.

Instead of encouraging them to finish what's on their plates, ask them questions like:

> ✔ Check in with your fullness level. Are you sure you've had enough?
>
> ✔ Notice how much food you've left. Can you start out with less next time?
>
> ✔ Have you had enough of this food and are you perhaps hungry for something else?

Teaching children about being mindful of waste is okay. As adults, we can do that without making them feel guilty. Children often take more than they can eat when their eyes are bigger than their stomachs. Simply remind children to take less and let them know that they can always go back for more if they're still hungry.

Parents also commonly serve their children portions based on what they think is an appropriate amount for their children to eat, and sometimes this can be hard to accurately judge.

As soon as your children are old enough, encourage them to serve themselves while you act as a supporting guide, helping them to get better at choosing an adequate amount of food. Children can then get used to checking in with how hungry they are and portioning out food appropriately.

As a parent, remind children that when they've finished what's on their plates, they can pause for a few moments and check in with their hunger and fullness again. If they're still hungry they can always go back for more food. Again, help them portion out a second serving, guiding them based on your best judgment of an adequate amount of food.

Being patient with picky eaters

Children can be picky eaters. Sometimes, inevitably, children won't like a particular meal that their parents are serving. Understandably, dealing with picky eaters on a daily basis is frustrating for parents.

However, when a child claims to dislike a food, his or her opinion is quite valid. Even as adults, we all have likes and dislikes related to food.

Keep in mind that children's pickiness can and oftentimes does change over time as children's food preferences shift and develop. Patience is essential in these situations. Don't make children feel bad because they don't like a food.

Instead, explore what they don't like about it by asking them questions like:

- How do you think we can prepare this food differently in ways that you may like?
- What do you think we can add to this food that may influence the way you like it?

You can also zero in on the specific senses to explore what it is exactly about this food that the child doesn't like.

- Is it the taste you don't like?
- Is it the smell?
- Is it the temperature?
- Is it the texture?
- Is it the way it looks?

Invite your children to experiment. Ask them, 'Would you like to have fun and play with your food?' Ask them to close their eyes and smell their food. Ask them to describe the smell. Then ask them to take a bite with their eyes closed and describe to you what it tastes like. Do they still not like it?

Children often have to try the same food numerous times, prepared in various ways, before they begin to like it. Keep playing with new ideas and invite them to be active participants in the process. Avoid labeling your children as picky eaters, unless of course, you want it to become a self-fulfilling prophecy!

In the past few decades, the number of children dealing with food-related allergies has skyrocketed. Often allergies can be hidden and manifest in symptoms like an upset stomach, headaches, bloating, gas, diarrhea and so on. If children are intuitively not eating a food, they may have good reasons. Be open and trust what your children have to say. Explore your children's concerns with a genuine attitude so that they feel empowered and can listen to what their bodies are saying to them.

Including children in meal selection and preparation

To help encourage children to cultivate a positive relationship with food, include them in the activities that surround eating, not only the act of eating itself.

Involving children in grocery shopping, meal preparation and clean up gives children a sense of appreciation for all that goes into placing a meal on the table. They gain a stronger connection to where their food comes from and discover how to feed themselves healthfully, acquiring the skills that they need as they enter adulthood.

Grocery shopping

These days, taking children into grocery stores, which are stocked with brightly colored packages designed to attract children's attention, can be challenging. Educating your children about real, whole foods becomes of prime importance. You may or may not decide to take them into conventional grocery stores with you; however, think about other ways you can include your children in the grocery-shopping process.

If you do decide to venture into the large commercial grocery stores, use the visit to educate your children about the difference between real, whole foods and packaged foods. Try to focus on the periphery of the store where the fresh foods are sold and avoid the middle aisles.

Alternatively, farmers' markets are wonderful places to bring your children. These days, more and more local farmers' markets are popping up all over the world, especially in the summer time. These markets are a great way to teach your kids about the benefits of eating locally grown, organic food and make a connection with the people who you're buying from. In addition to farmers' markets, you may also want to bring your kids with you to shop at food co-ops or local health food stores.

Meal preparation

Including your children in the process of preparing a meal teaches them invaluable skills and has a major impact on the way that they nourish themselves for the rest of their lives. You also experience fun quality time spent together, and you get the opportunity to educate them about healthy eating. You may also notice that including children in meal preparation gives them a sense of personal responsibility and ownership over the process and may result in less picky eating, even amongst the pickiest of eaters! Ask them for their input and give them the option to make decisions: 'Would you rather have cucumber or celery for the dip?' or 'Would you rather have a blueberry or a raspberry smoothie for breakfast?'

You can invite children to:

- ✔ Wash produce
- ✔ Stir or mix a batter
- ✔ Toss a salad
- ✔ Set the table
- ✔ Sprinkle a seasoning
- ✔ Measure out ingredients

As children get older and slowly gain more experience, increase their responsibility in the kitchen. Take turns and shift roles. Ask your child to plan out a meal and support and guide them in the process. Make meal-planning fun with themed meals like Taco Tuesday, Mexican Fiesta or Roll Your Own Sushi night.

Teaching children about some of the potential dangers in the kitchen is extremely important. Educating children about sharp knives, hot stoves and avoiding fingers in blenders is essential. Teaching kids to move with mindfulness and attention is crucial for their safety and well-being.

Meal clean-up

Cleaning up after a meal doesn't have to be boring or feel like a chore. Make clean up more enjoyable by:

- ✔ Playing music and have a sing-along in the kitchen while putting the dishes away.
- ✔ Playing a game to determine who will do the dishes after a particular meal.
- ✔ Make two teams with separate tasks and see who can complete their tasks first. (Scoring can also include how well the job was done.)

If parents always clean up after their children, kids learn that they don't have to take responsibly for their contribution to the mess. Inviting everyone to at least wash their own dish, utensils and glassware is a great place to start.

Setting a mindful example

Educating children about healthy dietary habits can be quite challenging in today's food environment. Parents carry a lifetime of belief systems around food. Ultimately parents can only do the best they can and teach their children what they think is best for them.

Allowing children the freedom to decide what their food-related belief systems are is important. If you're a vegetarian parent, how will you handle the issue if your child wants to explore eating meat? If you serve meat at every meal, how will you handle it when your child wants to try vegetarianism? As parents, supporting dietary experimentation is important as it encourages the process of self-discovery and allows children to grow up with self-confidence.

When educating children about particular foods, avoid referring to foods as 'good' or 'bad'. Doing this sets children up to look at food from an all-or-nothing mentality and can put bad foods on a pedestal of desire. Children often want what they're not allowed to have, so educating kids about the difference between healthy and less-than-healthy choices is beneficial. Essentially, children need to make their own choices, and what you can do as a parent is to inform them of the consequences of their choices.

Consider raising children in a healthy food environment where special snacks and treats are only consumed on rare occasions in a mindful manner. Avoid using dessert as a reward by saying things like, 'If you want to eat dessert, then you have to finish your dinner.' When you do, dinner appears less than enjoyable, and something that must be consumed only to get something better.

Mindful eating exercises for children

This chapter is sprinkled with various mindful eating exercises that you can engage in with your family and your children. Here are two more formal mindful eating exercises that you can play with your kids.

Fruit from outer space

This is a fun and playful exercise that you can play with your children to not only encourage them to eat more mindfully, but also to get them excited about exploring new foods.

For this mindful eating exercise, you have to find an interesting-looking exotic fruit – a fruit so interesting looking that you could almost believe that it came from outer space. Regular grocery stores are increasingly stocking more exotic fruits. If you live in a city, explore your local China Town or Asian markets and try to find the most interesting-looking fruit. You may even want to include your kids in this stage and make it part of their exploration of discovering new foods. Some examples of interesting-looking fruit include: dragon fruit, passion fruit, star fruit, atemoya, jackfruit, pineapple, papaya, kiwi fruit and persimmon. Try to pick up a couple of different fruits to experiment with, just in case one of your kids has a strong aversion to one of the chosen fruits.

Ask your kids to explore this fruit with all of their senses and follow the script of the introductory mindful eating exercise provided in Chapter 9, and then if you like, follow up with the 'last bite of your life' exercise in the same chapter.

Ask your kids to describe what that experience was like. Ask them what they learned, what they liked about the fruit and what they didn't like.

Permission to play with your food

One of the best things you can do is to encourage children to have fun and be playful. Give kids permission to play with their food and eat in whatever way feels comfortable for them. It's okay if children want to eat with their hands and fingers. They can experience their meal differently and perhaps more enjoyably. People from many cultures in the world never actually use utensils, but eat with their hands their whole lives. Allow kids to be kids! We have a lot to learn from them when it comes to mindful eating.

Chapter 11

Mindful Eating in Social Situations

*Y*ou are a social being by nature, and eating with others is one of the primary ways that you connect with other people. These days, almost all social situations seem to revolve around food. Holidays, work parties, sporting events, you name it – food is involved. In our culture, food has become one of the primary methods of social entertainment. Given that almost all social activities are associated with eating, you need to discover how to navigate these situations more mindfully to prevent yourself from falling into the trap of mindless eating.

The Challenge of Eating Mindfully in Social Situations

This strong correlation between socializing and eating does not bode well for the many people who struggle with mindless eating, overeating or making healthy food decisions when unhealthy food options predominate.

Eat, drink and be merry: Avoiding feeling awkward at social events

Do you feel challenged by eating at social events because you eat differently than most other people? Maybe you're a vegetarian, vegan, raw foodie or are simply health conscious and don't like to eat foods that are not whole foods or organic. You can feel awkward attending a social event without having access to anything that you feel appropriate to eat, especially when people start asking questions like, 'Why aren't you eating that?'

Here are a few tips to help you navigate questions like these:

✔ **Share openly:** If people are asking, and you feel comfortable sharing with them, let them know why you're choosing or not choosing to eat something, whether it's for health, mindfulness or other reasons.

✔ **Respond with a question:** Ask them in turn why they eat the way they do.

✔ **Doctor's orders:** Politely let them know that your doctor or nutritionist has advised you to not eat certain foods for health reasons.

✔ **Change the subject:** Next time you feel uncomfortable about a food situation, take the pressure off by changing the subject.

Social pressure to conform should not be underestimated, and you may feel like you have to conform to the often unhealthy meals of the standard western diet. One thing you can do is to plan ahead by eating beforehand or bringing a healthy dish with you to share with others and have for yourself.

Remember that by choosing to eat healthily, you're setting a good example for others!

If you tend to overeat while eating with others, you're not alone. Almost everyone is prone to consuming more than they normally do while in the presence of other people. This overeating tends to happen for many reasons:

✔ **Social Influence**: You look to others as an indication of what is a socially acceptable amount to eat. If other people keep eating throughout the whole social event, then you recognize that behavior as socially acceptable, and you give yourself permission to do the same.

> ✔ **Emotions:** You may eat because you feel nervous, excited, bored, or any other uncomfortable emotion that you're trying to distract yourself from with food.
>
> ✔ **Distraction**: You may be distracted by conversations and continue to eat or overeat without paying attention, leading to mindless eating.

Although these situations can be tricky to navigate, if you're up for the challenge, you can gain insight into your relationship with food from these experiences. What's required is that you approach these social situations with mindful awareness, curiosity and a strong willingness to have self-compassion, because, inevitably, you'll catch yourself having mindless moments.

Hopefully, with a continued dedication to mindful practice, these moments become increasingly infrequent, and you can mindfully enjoy social events without having to worry about the negative consequences of mindless eating.

Don't Miss Out on the Fun: Eating at Social Events

We all crave social connection and seek companionship and time shared with friends and family. For some, social events are challenging to navigate, especially when they revolve around food. Incorporating mindful eating in social situations can be a rocky road at first. You'll undoubtedly face tricky situations that make eating mindfully a challenge.

Remember that you can enjoy special social occasions in a mindful way without feeling guilty about it.

You can bring three specific easy to implement and easy to remember mindful eating skills with you into any kind of social situation. You can add these tools to your mindful eating tool belt. (Check out Chapter 8 for the five basic mindful eating tools.) If you can focus on practicing and getting better at these three skills, you're well on your way to paving a more mindful path.

Doing one thing at a time

One of the most challenging parts of eating mindfully in social situations is the constant distraction away from eating. Our primary distraction at social events is . . . you guessed it – *socializing!*

The next time you're at a social event, try to remember this very simple instruction:

When you eat, simply eat and when you socialize, simply socialize.

To help you become more mindful of what, how and why you're eating, stick to doing one thing at a time. Trying to get as many things done at once as possible is deemed a good skill to have in our culture. However, when you do multiple things at once, you don't fully appreciate or experience each of the activities that you're engaging in.

The next time you're at a social gathering with food, make a conscious effort to separate your socializing and conversations from your eating.

If you're holding a plate of food or sitting at a table eating and someone starts a conversation with you, you can respond in one of two ways:

- ✔ Put down your fork or eating utensil, pause, take a breath in and then shift your attention to the conversation.

- ✔ If you prefer to eat and not converse at that moment, politely let that person know that you'd like to finish your meal and when you're done you'd love to have a conversation with him or her.

Be mindful of the type of conversation that surrounds a meal. When your conversation is focused on a very negative topic or surrounds intense emotions, the way you experience your meal can be influenced and make it less enjoyable.

Try this people-watching experiment the next time you're at a social gathering to gain insight into your mindful (or mindless) eating habits. The great thing about social events is that they make for wonderful people-watching opportunities. Just sitting back and observing how people engage with food from a non-judgmental perspective can be extremely valuable. The simple act of observing others is a very useful mindfulness tool, and you can gain deep insight into the way you choose to engage with your food.

The next time you're at a social gathering, take a moment to pause and simply observe. If you're at a serve-yourself event, after you're seated, take a moment to observe other people before you start eating. What do you see? Try to notice the different ways people are engaging with their food. Also pay attention to what it feels like to slow down your own eating process.

Perhaps you see friends eating really fast, talking while they eat and barely chewing before swallowing. Maybe you recognize some of these patterns of eating in yourself and observing it from an outside perspective, without judgment, helps you to be aware of your own mindless eating.

Pausing before you eat

Getting swept up by the commotion of any kind of social event is easy. The simple act of pausing before you eat completely changes the way you proceed to eat a meal and tunes you back into the present moment. Pausing only takes a few moments and is an essential technique to help you set the tone for mindful eating in any social situation.

You can use a mindful pause before mealtimes in any number of ways:

✔ Take a few deep breaths before eating.

✔ Take a moment to connect to your inner body awareness by doing a quick body scan (Chapter 8 has information on how to do a body scan).

✔ Notice any emotions you may be feeling.

✔ You may want to say a food blessing in silence.

✔ Use this pause to notice if you're being triggered to eat because of any number of social or environmental cues that may prompt a mindless overeating episode. (Go to Chapter 3 to find out about mindless eating triggers.)

> ✔ Observe other people's eating behavior, as described in
> the people-watching experiment earlier in this chapter.

You can also use a momentary pause during a meal as a
reminder to ask yourself if you're still hungry or getting full.
Using the hunger-fullness scale described in Chapter 8 can be
useful here.

Instead of just getting up for a second helping, pause and ask
yourself, 'Why am I getting more food right now? Am I still
hungry? Am I eating because everyone else is eating?'

If you're feeling really distracted, you may want to excuse
yourself from the table and go somewhere private like the
bathroom or step outside for some fresh air and have a
moment alone to check in. Take a moment to close your
eyes and feel your body from the inside out, perhaps running through a quick body scan, as described in Chapter 8.
By taking a moment to reconnect and get grounded, you can
prevent yourself from being swept away by the commotion of
a social event.

Noticing your triggers

Social events are rife with triggers to eat and overeat. Look at
Chapters 3 and 13 for more about food triggers and explore
what your most common triggers are in social situations.
After you have awareness of your triggers, you're in a position
to create new choices for yourself.

Make a list of your top three triggers in social situations.
How can you remind yourself to pay attention to these cues?
In what ways can you create a back-up plan the next time
you're being triggered? Visualize yourself being triggered and
responding rather than *reacting* to the situation. What new
choice do you make? What does it *feel* like to make this new
choice? Write down your answers in your mindful eating journal (see Chapter 4 for more on starting a journal).

Choosing Wisely: Eating in Restaurants

In the US, the average person spends almost half of their food dollars in restaurants. Not only do people eat out in restaurants to celebrate, for business meetings and as a matter of convenience, but also just for something to do.

Preparing meals at home is more supportive of a healthy lifestyle as you have more control over the quality of the ingredients and quantity of the portion sizes. Restaurants often make their foods taste *hyperpalatable*, that is, exceptionally good, by increasing the sugar, fat and salt content of their food. This flavor boost often overrides our natural, inherent ability to stop eating when we're full and prompts us to overeat, which is easy to do considering the ever-increasing portion sizes.

When you eat in restaurants, do you typically leave feeling overly full? What do you think your top three triggers that prompt you to mindlessly overeat in restaurants are?

Larger portion sizes have become the norm in restaurants. This situation is not ideal for the majority of people who have a hard time leaving food on their plates, despite how full they are. Here are a few suggestions to help you become more mindful of your food consumption in restaurants:

- ✔ Order an appetizer as your main meal.
- ✔ Share a main dish with someone else.
- ✔ Ask your waiter to bring you a to-go container with your meal and put half of your meal in there as soon as you receive it.
- ✔ Remind yourself that you don't have to clean your plate.
- ✔ Ask for sauces and dips on the side.
- ✔ Order exactly what you want, even if it's not on the menu, especially if you want to create a healthier option for yourself.
- ✔ Eat a healthy snack like a whole fruit before you go out to eat.

If you're dining out with a group or a friend, have a say in which restaurant you go to. Try to pick a restaurant that serves a variety of healthy foods, preferably with local and organic ingredients. Avoid buffets, fast-food restaurants and places with a limited selection.

Depending on the situation, try suggesting meeting over a cup of tea or going for a nice scenic walk instead of eating at a restaurant. Walk and talks are a great way to connect, especially for one-on-one business meetings. Eating during business meetings is best avoided, especially if stress is a foreseeable factor.

Proceed with Caution: Eating during the Holidays

The holidays are special occasions when you connect and share time with your loved ones. You gather with your immediate family, relatives and close friends to give thanks for your lives, your relationships and the sustenance from the earth.

Amongst all the joyful celebrations, the holidays can also trigger anxiety for people who struggle with food. The holidays tend to be food-centric as eating often takes center stage. That makes holiday gatherings prime territory for overeating and, of course, over-drinking.

When families come together they often carry emotional baggage from the past. Your family members can trigger you unlike anyone else. Dealing with challenging in-laws, childhood dramas between siblings or cousins, conflict between parents and their adult children can all trigger familiar emotional reactions, prompting you to numb out, avoid and distract with food. On the other hand, the holidays can also trigger fond childhood memories of connection, love and laughter, and you may associate holiday meals with the love you perhaps seek in your life. Whatever the case may be, strong emotional triggers often underlie the surface of holiday festivities and can influence your eating behavior.

Disrupting your typical routine

The holidays can also throw you off of your normal eating routine – late night dinners, potluck-style buffets, more snack foods at the workplace, holiday desserts and don't forget Grandma's baking! Simply being around more food can trigger you to eat more, let alone the constant social distractions and social acceptability of overeating during the holidays.

People often dread the upcoming holidays in fear of the additional weight that tends to go along with them. But you can enjoy the holidays without being consumed by constant thoughts of food and fear of weight gain.

Staying committed to mindful eating can be more challenging during the holidays – that's why the practice of self-compassion, as described in Chapter 5, is so important to keep in mind. Mindful eating takes practice, and social gatherings are rife with particularly strong cues towards overeating. Also remember that occasionally overeating during the holidays is not the end of the world, and it doesn't have to spiral you out of control. Be patient with yourself and don't give up!

Working with cravings

During the holidays, cravings to overindulge can be of particular concern. Being bombarded by so many tempting options can spiral anyone into a cycle of craving and desire. When you get swept up into the energy that comes with craving, resisting temptation becomes harder. Flip to Chapter 12 for a more thorough discussion on working with cravings, but for now, keep in mind that when you flex your mindfulness muscles you bear witness to cravings without being swept away by them.

During the holidays, pay particular attention to what may be triggering your cravings. Put on your detective's hat. If you shine a magnifying glass on your triggers and cravings, you immediately disempower them. Is it the sight of a table full of food? Is it the familiar holiday smells coming from the kitchen? Is it the people you're with? Is it particular emotions surrounding the holidays? Can you simply enjoy the sight and smell of food for what it is in this moment without amplifying a craving?

Minimizing mindless eating episodes

You can enjoy yourself and have a positive overall holiday experience without constantly being caught up in cravings and overindulging to the point of discontent. You're more prone to mindless eating when you're overtired, overstressed and overextended.

During the holiday season try to follow these simple suggestions:

- **Don't overcommit yourself:** Just because lots of holiday festivities are happening, you don't have to attend each and every one. Many people have FOMO – fear of missing out. Making enough time for yourself is important so that you don't feel overly stressed out with commitments.

- **Stay active and try to make a point of exercising once a day:** Exercising helps boost the feel-good chemicals in your brain, boosts your capacity for mindfulness and helps curb cravings.

- **Get enough sleep:** You often overextend yourself to the point of exhaustion during the holidays. Overeating can also result due to stress and fatigue.

- **Set intentions:** Set your intentions to pay attention, to make conscious choices around food and to commit to self-compassion if you forget to be mindful.

- **Use the power of visualization:** Picture yourself at a holiday gathering and imagine yourself making mindful food choices. Feel what it's like to stop eating before you're overly full and to make healthy food choices.

At holiday gatherings remember to:

- **Keep coming back to the present moment.** During the holidays, you have the pleasure of experiencing many delicious foods, but only if you're present to actually experience and taste them! Also stay present when you notice yourself worrying about upcoming meals or holiday gatherings.

- **Notice your emotions:** Pay particular attention to what thoughts and feelings arise. If you notice you're feeling nervous, excited or anxious, tend to those feelings before you decide to eat food.

✔ **Bring a healthy dish with you:** You may be faced with countless unhealthy dishes at holiday gatherings. Take the time to prepare a healthy alternative to share, like a salad, vegetable dish or fruit salad for dessert.

✔ **Avoid grazing:** Commit to eating a meal sitting down at a table to prevent yourself from constantly picking at food.

✔ **Bring a doggie bag:** To encourage yourself not to overeat, bring a container with you so that you can take leftovers home and enjoy the special holiday food again the next day.

✔ **Limit alcohol consumption:** If you struggle with overeating (and especially if you're driving), limit alcohol consumption. Alcoholic beverages have more calories than most people assume and can trigger you to overeat come mealtime.

On the Go: Eating Mindfully while Traveling

Traveling to new places with unique and unfamiliar food cultures is a wonderful way to explore mindful eating. Each meal offers you an opportunity to engage all your senses in an unfamiliar experience. Because you're not used to it, you tend to engage more mindfully as you explore unknown territory.

While traveling, you don't always have access to the healthy foods you are used to, but you can potentially explore new fruits and vegetables that you've perhaps never heard of. Simply do the best you can and enjoy the experience for what it is. Remember that you can adopt your regular eating routine when you arrive back home.

Planning ahead

Do a little bit of research about the place that you're visiting. Does your accommodation have a refrigerator? Is there a local market or grocery store where you can go shopping for your own food instead of having to eat out at every meal?

Happy, healthy and whole: Discovering great food options when you travel

When preparing for a trip, you can plan ahead by searching online listings for healthy restaurants in the place you're traveling to.

Websites like www.happycow.com have a directory of healthy restaurant and food store listings in almost every major city in the world. This particular website gives you many options, from vegetarian to vegan to raw food, and lets you know all the different types of foods that are available at each restaurant. The website provides customer reviews so that you can see what other people have to say about their experiences, and it also gives you the opportunity to write a food review of your own – a wonderful mindful eating exercise!

If you're traveling in the US or Canada, check out www.eatwellguide.org for a similar resource on finding local, organic and sustainably grown food.

Healthy travel tips

While traveling, remember to:

- ✔ Stay hydrated and drink plenty of clean, filtered water.
- ✔ Eat light foods that are easy to digest.
- ✔ Pack some healthy snacks with you.
- ✔ Avoid eating in fast-food restaurants.
- ✔ Explore that particular area's unique and unfamiliar fruits and vegetables.

Unfamiliar ethnic foods offer us rare sensory experiences. Use any of the practices outlined in Chapter 9 to develop your mindful eating skills, especially the practices inviting you to explore your five senses.

While traveling, be mindful of what, how and why you're eating; be gentle with yourself and kind to your body, and don't forget to have fun and enjoy your trip!

Chapter 12

Overcoming Obstacles to Mindful Eating

In This Chapter

▶ Exploring and working with strong cravings

▶ Discovering how to navigate a mindless eating slip-up

▶ Incorporating mindful eating into busy schedules

*D*eveloping mindfulness skills – like acquiring any new skill – takes time. On this journey you can expect road bumps and obstacles along the way. Just as when you're confronted with any obstacle in life, if you choose, these situations can provide ample learning opportunities. You can use these challenging times to deepen your understanding of your relationship with food and discover how to navigate your path with even more attentive precision.

As the famous saying goes: 'It's not how many times you fall down but how many times you get back up that counts.'

Working with Cravings

Sudden cravings and the seemingly unbearable desire to give in to temptation are undoubtedly some of the main obstacles that throw even the well-versed mindful eater off course. If you've ever experienced a strong craving for a particular food, you surely know what I'm talking about.

Cravings are usually associated with:

✔ **Automatic pilot:** Chances are that in the past, when you had a craving, you followed through on pursuing it until you satisfied that need. Sometimes you may not have been aware that a craving triggered you. (See Chapter 3 for more on cues and triggers to eat.) The more times you do this, the stronger the automatic pilot becomes and increases the chance that you'll mindlessly reach for something out of impulse (see cookie; eat cookie). When your focus is hooked on the craving, flexing your conscious decision-making mind can be challenging.

✔ **Irrational mind:** You can think of this as your 'inner saboteur'. This is the part of your mind that tells you anything that supports the attainment and satisfaction of your craving. It convinces you that pursuing this craving is a very good idea and in your best interest, and it defends whatever particular food you're craving down to the wire. It also tries to make you forget all the disadvantages of eating the cake, the cookie, the pizza and so on.

✔ **Severe restriction:** Constant dieting and restriction over long periods of time can understandably lead to cravings. Usually an equivalent and opposite binge offsets periods of restriction. You find yourself on a constant pendulum swing; after momentum is gained, stopping becomes harder and harder.

✔ **Desire to satisfy an emotional need:** Cravings can often have more to do with satisfying an emotional need than a physiological need.

✔ **A sense of stuckness:** When caught in the midst of a food craving, you often feel stuck in it.

✔ **Desire for a specific food:** When cravings strike they usually narrow in on very specific foods. These cravings are different from genuine hunger where a range of options is acceptable to satisfy your hunger.

✔ **Desire for foods high in sugar and fat:** Foods high in sugar and fat give you the most sensory pleasure and can have a strong impact on the feel-good chemicals in your brain, inducing a very powerful emotional response that you recognize as pleasure and feeling good.

✔ **A very sudden and urgent need or desire:** Cravings usually hook you very suddenly. You can go from a zero to a ten on the craving scale in a matter of seconds.

Take a moment to reflect on the foods that you crave. In your mindful eating journal, make a list of your top five foods. (Chapter 4 details how to start a mindful eating journal.) Have you always craved these foods or do you go through food phases? When do you typically crave these foods? Who are you with? What time of day is it? What feelings were you experiencing right before the craving?

You don't need to feel bad about your cravings. Everyone craves something from time to time. Most people label the foods they crave as bad and then label themselves as bad as well. Indeed, these food choices may not be the healthiest options, but give yourself a little self-compassion. You're biologically designed to seek out high-calorie foods. You have deeply rooted memories associated with the foods you crave, and these memories can have a very powerful effect on your behavior. You're also surrounded by these less-than-healthy hyperpalatable, high-calorie food choices at every turn. Over time, with continued dedication to get back up, navigating these food-craving situations becomes easier.

Becoming mindful of cravings

Mindful eating helps you navigate inevitable food cravings. With mindfulness you discover how to become unstuck or unhooked from your cravings. Oftentimes, you may feel that a craving is taking over your whole being. Mindfulness helps you to step back and look at your cravings for what they really are. In this process you reclaim your rational, curious and aware mind from your unconscious and irrational mind.

When you're being mindful of your cravings you have insights into the true nature of these feelings – namely, that they're transient, in motion and not as stuck as you believed.

Oftentimes, cravings are actually fueled by a storyline that you've created in your mind based on unexamined beliefs and perceptions. Some of these mistaken thoughts may include the belief that:

- The food you desire will bring you relief from pain.
- The food will bring you lasting pleasure.
- You like the food that you're craving.

✔ The food will allow you to avoid something that you have to do eventually.

✔ The food will prevent you from feeling something that you don't want to feel.

Essentially, when you crave, you're looking outside of yourself for something to bring you happiness. As Eastern wisdom traditions teach, this path inevitably only leads to more suffering. What follows are a number of suggestions to help unhook yourself from food cravings.

Feeling into it

Is it possible that you can become more mindful of your thoughts and emotions that may be fueling a craving? The following 'feeling into it' technique allows you to get out of your thinking mind and into your feeling body by noticing the story line of thoughts surrounding a craving and then connecting to the underlying energy that you're actually feeling in your body.

The next time you catch yourself in the middle of a food craving, take a moment to pause and notice what thoughts are going through your mind. Then move your awareness from your mind into your body. What do you physically feel? Try to describe the sensation: Is it hot? Cold? Pulsing? Overwhelming? Nervous? Excited?

This practice allows you to become more mindful of what you're actually physically experiencing – an excellent mindfulness tool in its own right, and one that can loosen the tight grip that thoughts often have during a craving episode. Try experimenting with coupling this exercise with the next one, 'surfing the urge', for even better results.

You may also want to use this in conjunction with the body scan outlined in Chapter 8 as a supporting relaxation technique.

Surfing the urge

One of the potential consequences of cravings is that you can get lost in them. You feel overtaken and swept up by the often intense or overwhelming energy that can accompany cravings. As a result you can self-identify with the craving rather than seeing it for what it is – a transient, impermanent, fleeting state of mind. A craving does not define who you are. The following mindfulness technique called 'surfing the urge' helps you to see that cravings simply come and go and helps you observe this effect happening without the need to get lost in it or identify with it.

The next time you're experiencing a craving, tune into the energy you're feeling in your body, as described earlier in the section 'Feeling into it'. If you feel overwhelmed by this energy visualize yourself in the ocean. Imagine that a wave is coming your way and you're ready to catch it on your surfboard. When you feel a welling up of underlying energy, grab your board and ride it out like a wave. Explore all the sensations that you're feeling. When you shine the light of awareness on a food craving, you notice the transient, changing nature of cravings; just like the waves in the ocean, eventually, they pass. In the end you see that you always have a choice: you can ride out the craving and feel the exhilaration of all the underlying sensations or you can get tossed and turned by the wave until you become exhausted and are swept up to shore.

Keeping a record of your cravings

One way that you can work with your cravings is to sit down and write about them in your mindful eating journal.

Keeping a record in the midst of a craving can be beneficial, but understandably, you may also find it challenging to do. Journaling about your craving after it's passed, no matter what outcome you chose to pursue, can also be very insightful.

The next time you're craving something, encourage yourself to grab your journal and a pen and explore the following questions:

- ✔ What is it you're craving?
- ✔ Where are you?
- ✔ What time of day is it?
- ✔ Who are you with?
- ✔ What were you feeling just before your craving started? (Tired? Stressed? Upset? Nervous?)
- ✔ What is the underlying energy you're feeling in your body?

> ✔ How would you feel afterwards if you pursued your craving?
>
> ✔ If you've already satisfied your craving, ask yourself how you feel now you've pursued your craving?

You can also experiment with combining journaling with any of the other exercises previously explained in this chapter for potentially better results. Find the methods that work best for you.

Tuning in properly: Do you really like that food?

As you start to eat more mindfully, you may notice that the story you were telling yourself about a particular food you crave isn't actually providing you with an experience that matches that long-held storyline. Working mindfully with food cravings invites you to notice how your mind is working and reminds you to tune into your body to strengthen your capacity to eat based on internal hunger cues.

I've seen the following scenario play out many times: when people start paying attention while eating the foods they *thought* they were craving, they realize that they don't even enjoy them! To my own amazement, I've experienced this situation myself; it was quite an eye-opening experience. Mindful eating tunes us into what we're *actually experiencing* as we slowly let go of our mind-constructed thoughts and stories *about* what we're eating.

For example, you may have a love-hate relationship with a particular food, say crackers and cheese. Within your particular food-related belief system, crackers and cheese are on your list of forbidden foods. When you're on the wagon you don't touch crackers and cheese, when you're off the wagon you engage in guilt-ridden consumption of them. Your labeling of this food as 'forbidden' also fuels your desire for it. However, if you were to drop the story line about the crackers and cheese and sit down to a direct experience of eating a single cracker and a single slice of cheese, what you notice may surprise you. You may experience this bite of food as a big blob of dryness in your mouth, sucking the moisture out of your mouth and leaving it parched and pasty. You may notice that the food's saltier than you had previously realized. You may notice that dairy foods give you a sore stomach, which you hadn't previously paid attention to because after you ate the crackers and cheese you were completely lost in self-critical thoughts. You may notice that what you've been *thinking* about the crackers and cheese isn't aligning with how you're actually experiencing the food.

Developing awareness: Pleasant, unpleasant and neutral

Try this essential mindful eating tool called 'pleasant, unpleasant and neutral' to bring awareness to your actual experience of a craving episode.

The next time you experience a strong desire to eat a particular food, give yourself permission to proceed slowly with mindfulness. Take your first bite and ask yourself: 'Is this experience pleasant, unpleasant or neutral?' Let go of whatever storyline you've created around this food and notice what your actual experience of it is here and now. Is it as amazing as you hoped it would be? Try to maintain a non-judgmental, open and curious attitude, and again ask yourself, 'In this moment, is this experience pleasant, unpleasant or neutral?'

You may also realize that just because your mind knows that it likes a particular food, it doesn't mean that your body always wants to eat it. Sometimes you may be ignoring a very clear signal from your body not to eat something, but the mental storyline is so strong it overrides your feeling-body awareness.

Finding the middle way when 'I really do like that food!'

Discovering that you don't actually like the experience of eating pizza, chips and ice cream may be a wonderful revelation, but what about when you really do like it? You check in and you feel confirmed that both your thoughts and your sensory experience is pointing to a resounding A+ on the pleasure scale. After all, these hyperpalatable foods are created to push all of our biological buttons to want, crave and desire them. Mindful eating comes in especially handy in this situation.

You can take a number of approaches when you find yourself in this scenario, but exploring what works best for you is important. Some strategies, if not appropriate for you, may backfire or set you up for an overeating episode. Use your best judgment and implement the strategies that you think are best for you.

One mindful bite

As you may know from personal experience, food restriction and being overly controlling of food intake can lead to food cravings and potentially to overeating episodes.

Can you satisfy your craving with one mindful bite? Or a small portion size? If you are the type of person who has a difficult time allowing yourself to have a small amount without polishing off the whole pint, bag or package, you may want to try the 'out of sight, out of mind' method described later in this chapter.

If you want pizza, instead of getting wrapped up in the craving for it, consider allowing yourself to have a single slice. Try to have only one condition: *that you will be present for the experience.* Discovering how to have one mindful bite can be more pleasurable and more satisfying than eating a whole pizza mindlessly. Try to eat slowly and without distractions (Chapter 8 has more on removing distractions). Also, be present for the entire experience, including how you feel afterwards. When you're fully present with what you're feeling afterwards you may decide that eating the pizza isn't actually worth it. And, when you're fully present for the experience of eating the pizza, you may notice that one slice is all that you need to feel satisfied.

Mindful eating is not about deprivation, it's about awareness. If you want to eat something, then the least you can do is to be fully present to experience it!

The 'first bite awareness' exercise where you fully engage all your senses while slowly eating a single bite of food is excellent for becoming mindful of your food cravings. (Flip to Chapter 9 for more details). Explore this mindful eating exercise with a food that you crave or perhaps struggle with in some way. Really try to pay attention to if the food maintains its pleasurable taste throughout the experience or if the third or fourth bites start to lose some of that taste sensation from your taste buds habituating to the taste. Try to pinpoint at which exact bite your taste satisfaction and enjoyment starts to decline. What did this experience teach you? Do you feel like it was helpful to become more mindful of taste when working with a craving?

A healthier option

Can you replace your craving with a healthier snack? If you're craving something sweet, can you turn to a wholefood option instead to satisfy that craving? Many fruits are especially sweet. Maybe you can make yourself a blueberry smoothie, eat a few figs or have some other kind of fruit. If you're in the mood for something creamy, why not make yourself a salad with a creamy salad dressing?

This practice of eating a healthy alternative can also backfire. Check out if this is a suitable approach for you. You may find it appropriate in some situations and not in others, so use your best judgment. Sometimes, when people try to avoid their cravings they eat everything else in sight and still crave what they initially wanted. They may still eat the food they were craving, plus all the other food eaten beforehand! Ask yourself if turning to a wholefood option is too restricting for you and if you would be better off eating what you actually want in a smaller portion size and in a mindful manner.

If you've eaten and you're no longer physically hungry but you're still craving a specific food, you have a prime opportunity to ask yourself what you're really hungry for. What nourishment can you give yourself that doesn't involve food?

Ask yourself to describe what it is that you're craving and go for the healthiest option that you feel satisfied with. You can also have a back-up plan in place and make a list of all the foods that you genuinely like that you can have as healthier options for your craving. These substitutes can be your go-to foods in times of need.

Out of sight, out of mind

For some people, managing cravings for specific foods is made easier by not keeping them in the house. By minimizing exposure you may prevent craving episodes. However, this option doesn't address how you manage your cravings when you inevitably encounter these foods out in the real world. Practicing the 'feeling into it' and 'surfing the urge' techniques described earlier in this chapter, as well as keeping a record of your cravings in your mindful eating journal, can be beneficial to you in these situations.

Taking care of yourself

Most of the time cravings arise due to an unmet emotional need. Look at how you can nourish yourself in other ways instead of with food. Take time to tend to your emotional needs and manage stress. Do a body scan, where you systematically bring your awareness to each part of your body, starting with your left foot and working your way through your whole body. (See Chapter 8 for a more detailed explanation.) It's an excellent tool to help you tune into what you're feeling and also to help you relax. Engage with friends, go for a walk and get outside in nature. Any activity that makes you feel good can help you to manage cravings.

Using the hunger-fullness scale

One way to increase your chances of cravings is to let yourself get extremely hungry. If you're chronically depriving yourself or if you're not paying attention to your hunger levels, you may be setting yourself up for a cycle of craving and/or binging. Try to have a back-up plan. Carry fruit with you or a few nuts or seeds for when you notice yourself getting really hungry or when you're in a situation where you can't get food. Don't let yourself get to a 1 or 2 on the hunger-fullness scale, which is described in Chapter 8.

Getting Back on Track: Lapse and Relapse

Developing a new habit takes time. In the process of working toward establishing lasting, positive change, you can almost certainly expect to experience ups and downs along the way. As with any undertaking, experiencing three steps forward, one step backwards is not uncommon. Mindful eating for weight loss is not usually a linear process where you continuously lose weight until you reach your ideal realistic weight.

Try not to let every little slip-up completely throw you off the path. Self-sabotage can enter the picture and turn little, no-big-deal situations into unnecessarily larger ones. The path of mindful eating takes time, and establishing change takes time; be patient with yourself.

Because you can expect obstacles along the way, fostering a strong and positive mindful eating attitude, as outlined in Chapter 5, is important so that you can meet these times with compassion, acceptance and understanding.

The 'what the heck' effect

Have you ever eaten a single cookie only to convince yourself that you're a complete moral failure and then proceeded to eat the entire box? Whether to that extreme degree or lesser, almost everyone can identify with this all-or-nothing mentality that leads to the 'what the heck' effect trap. You eat something, you feel bad about it, and then you turn to more of that food to make yourself feel better. When you look at it with your rational mind you can see how illogical it is to think that way, yet many people continue to do it, in one way or another. That's the way your irrational inner saboteur tricks you into giving in, giving up and throwing your goals out the window.

One of the best ways to work with these situations and prevent yourself from spiraling out of control is by being kind, gentle and self-compassionate. Although it may sound counterintuitive, and you may be thinking this is just the right time to get stricter with yourself, research has shown that being overly strict will more likely prevent you from reaching your goals and further inhibit your motivation. Self-compassion, on the other hand, will help you put down the cookie and back away from the box without getting swept up in harsh self-critical thoughts. Remember, be your own best friend in times like these.

When was the last time you experienced this 'what the heck' effect? Do you think next time you can simply eat the cookie without feeling bad about it and needing to eat the whole box?

Paying attention: Every moment is a new moment

The power of mindfulness repeatedly teaches you that every single moment is a new moment. Although the concept of mindfulness is extremely basic – simply paying attention – what you can discover under the surface of that simplicity can be tremendously profound. All you have is this moment right now; nothing else exists.

As a human being, you're naturally inclined to want to resist change. But as the famous saying goes, 'The only thing that stays the same is change.' Even though you know that everything is constantly changing on an intellectual level, feeling

Letting go of the past

One rainy evening, two monks were returning to their monastery. As they were walking, the monks came upon a beautiful young woman who was standing in front of a deep puddle of water, unable to cross the road. The elder of the two monks went up to her and carried her to the other side of the road before continuing on his way to the monastery.

In the evening the younger monk came to the elder monk and said, 'Sir, as monks, we cannot touch women, and I saw you lift that woman up across the road.'

The elder monk smiled and answered, 'Yes, brother. I left her on the other side of the road, but it seems you are still carrying her.'

Remember this story when you are struggling with letting go of the past. Are you still carrying it around with you unnecessarily?

emotionally at ease with it is more difficult. Realizing that nothing stays the same is hard, as well as knowing that one day your own life will pass. Thinking about your life cycle in this way is not morbid or negative or depressing. Consider it as a great inspiration to wake up to your life and live it fully in the now!

Every moment is a completely new moment and offers you a fresh opportunity to make new choices that influence the direction of your future.

You can choose to reflect on the past as a method of learning from your previous mistakes. Such reflections can be beneficial, constructive and supportive of the new decisions that you're cultivating for moving forward. Constantly dwelling on the past, however, can prevent you from living your life in the present moment.

Making mistakes: Blessings in disguise

Getting down on ourselves is so easy when we make mistakes – or what we perceive to be mistakes.

In order to prevent good/bad, right/wrong thinking surrounding your food choices, notice how you relate to the term 'mistake'. I use this term loosely here to apply to the *way* an act is committed, rather than the act itself. For example, the act of eating chocolate cake is not in itself a mistake. It may be a mistake for you if you eat it feeling guilty and know within yourself that eating it is going to cause you more suffering. Perhaps eating it is not a mistake if you eat the cake mindfully and truly enjoy it. Only you define what mistakes are for you, and even then, they don't have to be mistakes, only growth opportunities!

If you are willing to be mindful with a non-judgmental attitude, you can look at these mindless moments as blessings in disguise and use them to your advantage as a catalyst for change. These 'mistakes' offer you fresh opportunities to deepen your understanding of your relationship with food and provide you with ample insights to help influence your future decisions.

Forgiving yourself and moving on

Interrupting a cycle of overeating or binging or any habitual pattern you no longer want to see in your life can be really challenging. However, if you can accept the simple truth that this moment is a new moment and that what you just did is now in the past, you can forgive yourself and move on. Deeply accept whatever just happened with love, compassion and non-judgment and allow yourself the space to move forward without carrying guilt around with you like a weight around your neck. Dwelling on the past is just another way that you can miss out on experiencing the joys of the present moment.

Practicing self-compassion

If you catch yourself eating mindlessly or making food choices that don't support your health, you can view this as a wonderful opportunity to strengthen your capacity for self-compassion. Self-compassion is a much more effective approach for handling setbacks than self-criticism. Self-criticism actually makes it harder to forgive yourself and move on and instead can keep you locked in a negative feedback loop. Chapter 5 looks at ways of practicing self-compassion, an essential mindset to foster, especially during setbacks.

Mindful Eating for Busy Schedules

You may be wondering how you're ever going to find the time to practice mindful eating, especially with your already very busy schedule.

You'll be happy to hear that essentially, it doesn't take any more time to be mindful than it does to be mindless. You've already made time for eating, haven't you? The moment is still the same, except that in one scenario you're paying attention to what you're eating and in the other scenario you're not!

But as a result of mindfulness, you may start to notice yourself willingly slow down to take more time to experience being present for a meal. Adding a few extra minutes onto a meal may become a by-product of cultivating mindful eating.

All you're doing is reminding yourself to be present for your eating and fully experience what it is you're eating. Pausing before you eat to tune into your body, or pausing between bites to check in with your fullness, takes a relatively small amount of time. Consider how many hours you spend a day watching television, surfing the web or talking on the phone. Eating mindfully may naturally lead to you slowing down and adding a few extra minutes on to a mealtime, but isn't that worth it if it allows you to have a more fulfilling, enjoyable relationship with food? Would you rather taste the food you're eating or would you rather be stressed out thinking about the meeting you're going to after lunch?

Ask yourself what's really important to you. If I told you that I'd pay you a hundred dollars for every time you ate a meal mindfully, how do you think your level of attention and effort would change? Would you miraculously make time for mindfulness? We make time for the things we prioritize in our lives. You decide what those priorities are. Do your health, well-being and life enjoyment rank high up on that list? Do you think that making more time for mindful eating will bring more satisfaction into your relationship with food and with life in general? You may want to reflect on these questions by assessing your relationship with food.

Chapter 13

Feeding Your Emotional Hunger

· ·

In This Chapter

▶ Discovering why you eat when you're not hungry

▶ Applying mindfulness to emotional eating

▶ Exploring what you're really hungry for

· ·

*I*f you're like most people, you want to improve your relationship with food in one way or another, and this includes discovering a balance between eating when you're hungry and avoiding eating when you're not hungry – something that everyone does on occasions.

If you know that you repeatedly turn to food as your go-to crutch, this begs the more important question of *why* – why do you eat when you're not hungry? Because many people are triggered to eat as a reaction to an emotional response, finding out how to deal with your emotions directly is of prime importance. In this chapter, I explore the whys of overeating, with a focus on emotional eating, as well as exploring ways to deal with emotions head on rather than swallowing them down with food.

After you come to realize how often you turn to food despite a lack of hunger, you can start to ask yourself the bigger underlying question to all this, which is: 'What am I really hungry for?'

Are You Really Hungry?

Have you noticed that being overweight or obese is now more the norm than the exception? Over two-thirds of the American population falls into these categories, with Canada and the UK not far behind. Although obesity is a complex issue with many factors involved, one of the reasons for escalating rates of obesity is simply because many people tend to eat when they're not hungry and continue to overeat past fullness.

Grab your mindful eating journal and a pen. (Chapter 4 tells you how to create a mindful eating journal.) Take a moment to pause and reflect on these questions and jot down whatever comes to mind:

1. When was the last time you ate when you weren't hungry? What was the scenario? Was it at the office when you came in after lunch to see muffins and donuts on the counter that you just couldn't resist? Was it when you were feeling bored at home and decided to fix yourself up a snack just for something to do?

2. When was the last time you ate past fullness? Think of the last time you felt yourself getting stuffed, with feelings of guilt, shame and regret looming on the horizon, yet you couldn't stop. Was it at the buffet dinner with your friends? At your aunt's house for her birthday? Or at the big game this past weekend?

If you're like most people, you can identify with one, if not both, of these questions. It has likely happened to you in the past few days, and perhaps even today! If this is the case, you're in good hands – or should I say, you're holding a good book in your hands! Experimenting with the mindful eating techniques offered throughout this book helps you to uncover what's motivating you to eat (when you're hungry and when you're not) and aids you to develop a positive relationship with food that sets you on the path to good health and wellbeing.

Many people eat despite a lack of hunger. If you notice that you do, don't feel bad about it! Feeling bad, well, *feels* bad, and who wants that? Check out Chapter 5 to discover how a daily dose of self-compassion is better for you than self-criticism.

Ten Questions to Ask Yourself Before You Eat

One of the most important benefits of mindful eating is that it allows you a moment to pause and ask yourself if you're actually hungry or if you're about to eat for one of the other million reasons people eat – without being hungry. To help you tune in and identify what's really going on under the surface ('Yes, I'm truly hungry,' or 'I'm really stressed out and I need to eat to calm my nerves,') run through a few very important questions first. These questions are a great way to help you flick that conscious switch on in your brain, shining the light of awareness on what you're currently doing and putting you back in touch with your body.

When most of my clients start eating mindfully, they find that they need some crucial in-the-moment guidance to help steer them in the right direction; that is, snapping out of autopilot and into the driver's seat. Asking a series of self-inquiring questions is one way to help train yourself on the spot – that moment in time when you're feeling the impulse to eat and you have an important decision to make: to eat or not to eat.

I first created this list of questions many years ago when I was constantly struggling with mindless eating (and it still comes in handy!) and have since shared it with thousands of people. I recommend sticking this list on your refrigerator or writing it out on a cue card and carrying it around with you in your purse or wallet and glancing at it in times of need.

The ten questions to ask yourself before you eat are:

- ✔ On a scale of one to ten, how hungry am I? (Flip to Chapter 8 for a full description of the hunger-fullness scale.)

- ✔ Am I really hungry or am I just thirsty? (Many people are very dehydrated and mistake hunger for thirst.)

- ✔ Am I about to eat because I'm tired? (Maybe I should take a nap instead?)

- ✔ Am I about to eat because I'm lonely? (Maybe I should call a friend?)

✔ Am I using food to procrastinate? (Maybe I just need a real break; how about five minutes in the sun?)

✔ Am I about to eat because I'm bored? (What can I do that is truly fulfilling or entertaining?)

✔ Am I eating because I'm emotional, and I don't want to feel what I'm feeling, so I avoid, distract or numb out with food. (Look at the section 'Eating Your Emotions' later in this chapter.)

✔ Am I about to eat because other people are eating? (We tend to eat more around other people. Use a reminder to check in with your hunger levels and read Chapter 11 for information on practicing mindful eating with others.)

✔ Will I feel guilty after I eat this? (Ask yourself: is it really worth it if I'm only going to feel worse in about ten minutes?)

✔ What am I really hungry for? (Check out the section 'What Are You Really Hungry for?' later in this chapter.)

Self-inquiry is a powerful tool in your mindful eating tool belt. Use these questions (or any new ones that you come up with that are appropriate for you) as a way to help identify and uncover what's really going on for you under the surface of 'I want to eat this . . . *now!*'

When you start to gain more self-awareness, actually following through on change can still take time. Even if you notice that you just want to eat because you're tired and cranky and you decide to eat anyway, you are still taking a step in the right direction. Be patient with yourself! Mindful self-awareness is an unfolding process that takes time to get to the point where you're ready to not only see what you're doing, but also to act differently than you have in the past.

Why You Eat When You're Not Hungry

Now here comes the tougher part. Are you ready to start looking under the hood to do some of the dirty work (okay, not exactly dirty, more like slightly uncomfortable)? This step requires asking yourself the more difficult questions that are often hard to face up to – the ones that you may have been turning a blind eye to and ignoring for a long a time. These are the *why* questions that are worth finding some answers to.

Uncovering your inner *whys* (*why* do I keep turning to food when I'm not hungry and when I know it's not helping me?) may feel a little prickly at first, but you can do it. This process is like peeling back the layers of an onion until slowly but surely you get to the inner core – your inner truth that helps you heal your relationship with food and eat more mindfully. And as always, whenever you're working with onions, tears may be involved – welcome them in; these tears are releasing what no longer serves you.

 Take a moment to pause and reflect. Grab your mindful eating journal and jot down any thoughts that come to your mind when you read this question: *Why do I eat when I'm not hungry?*

Don't censor yourself at this point; just write down whatever comes to mind. There's never only one answer to this question. You may have many reasons, and some of them may not even make sense to you in this moment, but write them down anyway. This exercise is your starting point. Feel free to come back and add to this list at any time, as new experiences present themselves or as new insights come to you.

Exploring this question and continuously coming back to it gives you insight into your relationship with food. Remember, only you can uncover the answers to this question for yourself. And although you have to discover your own truth to really benefit and improve your relationship with food, some tendencies are common to everyone and may help give you some insight into why you (and the rest of us) tend to continuously eat when you're not hungry.

Seeking the Power of Pleasurable Distraction

One thing that I think most people can agree on is: *life isn't always easy*. Especially in today's world, you're pressured to perform, achieve and be super productive. You're operating at a faster pace than ever before, and, as a result, your health is paying the price. Many people have demanding jobs, experience high stress levels, don't get enough hours of sleep at night and struggle with a dependency on stimulants (say hello to your morning cup of coffee!) as a means to keep up with the ever-increasing demands of life.

Pleasure seeker by design

Mother Nature knew what she was doing. You're biologically designed to be a pleasure seeker. The reason that food tastes yummy, sex feels great and social connection brings a smile to your face is because it's Mother Nature's way of trying to ensure the survival of the species by giving you a hit of pleasure from these survival-based mechanisms. This hit of bliss tells your brain to repeat whatever you just did – as a matter of survival. Although human biology hasn't changed much, the world you live in has drastically shifted from the subsistence-level time of your ancestors. Now we are constantly and chronically surrounded by all sorts of stimulating pleasures, so this biological design has become something of a double-edged sword.

Eating, for example, stimulates the reward pathways and pleasure centers of the brain by releasing serotonin, dopamine and other neurotransmitters in the brain that make you feel good. You need a certain level of 'feel-good' on a daily basis to function well emotionally, mentally and physically. However, problems start to arise when food becomes your primary go-to when you need a pick-me-up and want to feel good.

You see, there are healthy pleasure fixes and less-than-healthy pleasure fixes, and some things like food can fall on either side of the equation. Watching a sunset, playing with your kids, walking in nature, getting some sunshine on your skin, exercising, spending time with a loved one, all these things give you a daily dose of the feel-good that everyone seeks. But today, a plethora of other things that are highly stimulating can trigger a hyper-response in the brain's pleasure center and jolt you with a quick, temporary high, followed by a longer term low. (Hello, addiction and dependence). Drugs and alcohol are the first of these that come to mind, but excessive shopping, playing video games, TV watching and gambling can also be a problem.

Eating a balanced diet with lots of fresh, whole foods is a great way to get your daily dose of feel-good (think sitting down to a bowl of the juiciest, reddest cherries you've ever seen). But on the other hand, eating processed junk food can trigger an abnormally strong feel-good response that makes you want to come back for more – despite a lack of hunger.

Given all the chaos of this fast-paced lifestyle, who wouldn't want to step out of this hectic reality and experience a moment of peace? But because life can be . . . well, a little challenging to say the least, what you tend to seek out in your moments of peace is actually a moment of pleasure – because ultimately, what everyone wants is to feel good, and activating a feeling of pleasure helps to achieve that.

When seeking such peace, you may turn to food as a means of pleasurable distraction for good reason. You live in an age where you have easy access to pleasure that melts in your mouth. Food activates a part of the brain that makes you feel good without you always being fully aware that this is what food's doing for you. (The sidebar 'Pleasure seeker by design' has more about this topic.)

You see, not only does food feed your hungry cells, but it also brings a daily dose of happiness into your life – quite literally. When you eat, feel-good brain chemicals get released and give you a sense of pleasure. Essentially, food offers you a moment to step out of the demands and pressures of life and into a little bubble of bliss – until of course, the bubble bursts, and you're right back at your desk facing the to-do list that you were hoping to escape a moment ago.

Eating Your Emotions

Turning to food when difficult emotions arise is quite common. You may occasionally use food to deal with emotions: *'I'm feeling sad right now, so I'm going to sit down and eat something enjoyable and be present with this food.'* But if you continuously turn to food to stuff down your emotions, habitual patterns (and often unhealthy ones) tend to develop. Instead of dealing with your emotions directly, you just sweep them under the rug and never address what's really going on. If you keep doing this over many years, you'll eventually notice that you have a problem. Now, not only are you avoiding dealing with your stress levels by eating, on top of that you're dealing with being 30 pounds overweight and having high blood pressure.

The result? Your suppressed emotions wreak havoc on your life. Ask yourself if turning to food for that moment of pleasure is actually bringing you the pleasure, soothing or comfort that you're looking for. Or is it causing you more harm and pain in the long term?

Noticing emotional triggers

The first step to working with emotional triggers is awareness. You can't really take any action unless you have the awareness to know what you're dealing with.

Noticing your emotional triggers is a very important step in beginning to eat more mindfully. If you can recognize when you're turning to food even though you're not hungry and are using food as a way to 'eat your emotions', then you can start to make better decisions for yourself – decisions that are aligned with your health goals rather than with self-sabotage.

Some emotional triggers that may urge you to turn to food when you're not hungry are listed below. As you read this list, reflect on how often you eat as a reaction to feeling any of these emotions and circle the top three emotions that tend to prompt you to turn to food as a way of dealing with them – or put off dealing with them. You may be triggered to eat because you feel:

- ✔ Afraid
- ✔ Agitated
- ✔ Angry
- ✔ Anxious
- ✔ Bored
- ✔ Depressed
- ✔ Disappointed
- ✔ Embarrassed
- ✔ Excited
- ✔ Grieving
- ✔ Jealous
- ✔ Lonely

- ✔ Nervous
- ✔ Resentful
- ✔ Sad
- ✔ Stressed out
- ✔ Tired
- ✔ Uncomfortable
- ✔ Upset
- ✔ Worthless

Take out your mindful eating journal and a pen. When was the last time you were emotionally triggered to eat? What emotion were you feeling? What was the sequence of events? How did it feel to eat in that moment? Did eating give you the desired effect for more than simply a moment? What else could you have done instead of eating that could have helped you in that moment?

Covering over the surface: distracting and avoiding

Feeling bad sucks, plain and simple. That's why you do what you can to avoid it. When you feel something you don't want to feel, or an emotion that you don't know how to handle, you may notice yourself immediately doing something else to fill in the space – to cover over that bad feeling that you'd rather not experience.

Essentially, you do whatever you can to move away from the present moment. You do this in one of two main ways, so that ultimately you don't have to feel what you feel:

- ✔ By distraction
- ✔ By avoidance

Whether you eat to distract or avoid, these are both just different ways or styles of moving away from the present moment.

Identifying the root cause

Did you catch that last sentence? I hope so, because although it may sound simple, it is incredibly profound. Over the years, the more I reflect on this simple truth, the more depth and insight I gain into my own relationship to food and mindful eating. I think it bears repeating:

Ultimately, underlying all emotional triggers is an unconscious desire to move away from the present moment.

This is the root cause of many present-day problems and is one of the foundational teachings of Buddhist philosophy. Mindfulness is all about coming back to the present moment, over and over again, because you're always 'leaving', so to speak. Add to this any sort of uncomfortable bad feeling, and you're likely catching the next express train out of here – that is, the present moment.

Many people use food this way: to avoid the here and now (feeling upset) and try to be somewhere else (the bliss-filled land of chocolate).

Can you dig it? Getting to the root of the problem

Many people use food as a coping mechanism to distract themselves from dealing with their underlying problems. Your unconscious self is just trying to protect you from feeling more pain.

If you've repeatedly turned to food to avoid directly dealing with painful, difficult emotions, you've now created another problem for yourself. This issue becomes a new layer of something to focus on and struggle with, which inadvertently covers over the root of the original problem, the one that you'd rather not deal with.

Because some people's underlying issues feel too emotion-ally difficult to work with, creating a new (perhaps less pain-ful) problem to get caught up in seems easier, and for many people that's the food or weight struggle. As hard as strug-gling with food, weight, overeating, eating unhealthily or losing those last 10 pounds or 100 pounds seems, all of these issues are just superficial ones created to avoid dealing with the real problems.

Dealing with food issues may not be pleasant either; you may give anything to drop this struggle with food, except for dealing with the root of the issue.

Food does so much more than nourish you physically; it also feeds you emotionally. You always have more going on under the surface than simply a desire to lose weight or improve your relationship with food.

Many people have been burying their old problems with food for so long that they don't even remember what the initial trigger was that urged them to turn to food as a coping mechanism in the first place. Instead, the struggle with food (and often weight) now takes center stage of their problems.

Stop running away: feeling what you feel

Facing your emotions head on may seem counter-intuitive, but it's actually better for you. Allow yourself to feel what you feel; welcome your emotions in and explore them with curiosity rather than try to push them away or stuff them down with food.

Curiosity is a very powerful tool that helps you manage and work with emotions in a more friendly and light-hearted way.

Why would you want to feel what you're feeling when what you feel is bad? I know, that's a lot of feeling! But look more closely at your emotions and you'll discover something that actually needs to be addressed with your loving attention. Through this process you receive more insight, clarity and understanding than you can ever imagine.

Facing your emotions is like finally facing the big scary monster in your closet. All these years you've been avoiding that monster, afraid of it, but when you finally build up the strength and courage to confront it, that monster's not there.

How do you challenge your private monster? I use a simple two-step technique that I like to call 'out of your mind and into your body'. Your emotions are fueled by your thoughts – the story-line that you've created about the particular situation.

This practice allows you to drop the story line and tune into what you're physically feeling. Find a quiet, comfortable place to practice this exercise.

1. **Out of your mind:** Close your eyes and bring your awareness to your thoughts. Notice your thoughts and visualize them as clouds passing by in an open, vast sky. With the clouds floating by, bring your awareness into your body.

2. **Into your body:** To help you get out of your mind, focus on feeling what you feel in your physical body. Take a moment to try to sit quietly and tune into your body. Take a couple of deep breaths. What does this emotion actually feel like physically? Is your heart pounding? Are you sweating? Does your stomach hurt? Does your heart feel heavy? Are you shaking? Does it feel hot, cold, warm, itchy or jittery? Focus on your breath. Remember, your breath is your anchor to the present moment. Think of it as home base. How are you breathing at this moment? Explore your body with child-like curiosity, welcoming in whatever physical sensation you're feeling.

Personal writing is a great way to reveal and uncover deeper insights and awareness. Take a moment to reflect on this exercise and keep track of what you notice by writing in your mindful eating journal.

Your emotions can't hurt you

Your mind and your body are inextricably linked. What you think and feel emotionally influences your body. Sometimes emotions can feel physically painful – a clenched stomach, a heavy heart or a feeling of tightness in your chest. But rather than trying to push away what you're feeling, instead bring your attention to explore the physical sensations of these emotions with awareness. If you can do this, you'll discover that you're not as stuck in these emotions as you think; the underlying energy of these emotions is always changing and flowing, and the more you explore them and go into them, the more easily they dissipate and loosen their grip on you.

And the really good news is that despite how hard it may be to feel something emotionally painful, your emotions can't actually hurt you. No emotion improves by pushing it away, and, in fact, pushing your emotions away only make matters worse because what you resist persists. Even though you're just trying to protect yourself from feeling bad, not addressing your emotional needs only creates more challenges in the long run.

Gaining strength and courage

Discovering how to feel what you feel is no easy task. Developing the courage and strength to consciously choose to dive into your emotion instead of diving into a bag of chips takes time. You've been training in running away from these emotions (and the present moment) for many years, but over time you'll gain the strength and courage to lift up that rug and clean out the piles of emotional dirt that are now causing you more problems than they're worth.

What Are You Really Hungry for?

You've started uncovering what's really going on under the surface of mindless eating by gaining awareness through self-inquiring questions, identifying emotional triggers and exploring some of the reasons why you eat when you're not hungry.

This now begs the bigger question: what are you really hungry for? What is it you're really seeking in this moment, and, more importantly, in the moments you're turning to food?

Fulfilling your heart's desire

As human beings, what most people long for is meaning and purpose in their lives. You experience *soul hunger*, a deep inner desire to live the life that you most want to live. You tell yourself that you can't live that life for any number of reasons and continue to go about your life despite hearing an inner calling that you long to follow. But that path, that inner knowing, is often not easy to heed. Although that path offers many rewards, stepping out of your comfort zone and into the great unknown can be challenging. Most people tend to stand in their own way and are the greatest block to their own success. This was definitely the case for me, until one day I decided to step out of my own way and really live the life of my dreams. (The sidebar 'Following my heart's path' has more of my personal story.)

Following my heart's path

I spent many years of my life struggling with a disordered relationship with food and mindless eating. Food was my coping mechanism to cover over the unhappiness and depression that I felt when working in the finance industry.

One day it struck me like a thunderbolt: this wasn't supposed to be my path, and, more importantly, I no longer had to continue to choose this as my path. My heart was hungry for more meaning, more adventure and more fun! I sold or gave away everything I owned, packed a backpack and set off around the world on the adventure of a lifetime. I didn't have all the answers (how I was going to pay for everything or where I would live or even sleep that night!), I just took one step at a time, having faith that I could do whatever my heart was guiding me to. I knew I was on the right path because I felt good in my mind, body and spirit. I had spent so many years of my life not feeling good that I didn't want to waste another day of my life.

This has led me to where I am now. I live in one of the most beautiful places in the world, the islands of Hawaii, doing the work that I love. Obviously it's not everyone's life path to drop everything and become a traveling gypsy, but the underlying message is the same: when you follow your heart path of good intention and you really listen to your inner calling, the universe shows up to support you in ways that you could never even dream of.

If someone had told me ten years ago that I'd be married to an incredible man, living near the ocean and doing the work that I love, I would never have believed them! All I did was take one step in the direction of my heart, and the rest took care of itself.

One of the reasons you look for pleasure in food is because you're not getting enough pleasure from your life!

Get out your trusty paper companion – your mindful eating journal – and a pen. Take the time to really pause and reflect as you ask yourself these meaningful life questions:

✔ Am I happy doing what I'm doing?

✔ If I had all the money in the world, what would I do?

✔ If I could wake up to any setting (mountains, ocean, rainforest) where would that be?

✔ If I knew I couldn't fail, what would I do?

✔ What have I always wanted to do, learn, study or try, but didn't because I was afraid of not being good enough?

Creating a vision board of the reality you want to create for yourself can also be a fun process. Start collecting images of anything that you want to show up in your life and make a collage with them on a poster board. If you can't find an image that represents what you want to create in your life, then draw it! This vision board can also include positive words or quotes, images of people, places or things. The sky's the limit! Be creative and have fun with this process. It's your *life* you're dreaming up here!

Experiencing the simple pleasures in life

When it comes to creating an enjoyable life, you can dream big *and* you can also learn to enjoy what's already in front of you. Mindfulness, including mindful eating, can help you connect with the miracle of the simple pleasures in life that are constantly unfolding before your very eyes.

If you mindlessly turn to food when you're not hungry, you're seeking out a pleasurable response in your brain. For many, food becomes the primary way that they seek out pleasure, but you can do many other things to get your daily dose of the feel-good brain chemicals that help you to function optimally in your life.

Here are a few suggestions to get you started:

✔ Take a walk in the park.

✔ Wake up early and watch the sunrise (but not if you're overtired and lacking sleep!).

✔ Sleep in and read the paper in bed.

✔ Take a vacation.

✔ Play a game with your kids.

✔ Find more reasons to laugh!

✔ Don't take yourself too seriously.

✔ Plan a two-day road trip.

✔ Go for a picnic with a loved one.

✔ Volunteer in a place that needs some extra assistance.

✔ Go for a massage.

✔ Post notes with positive quotes and affirmations around your house.

✔ Curl up with a good book on the couch with a cup of tea.

✔ Spend more time in nature.

✔ Write in your journal.

✔ Learn a musical instrument.

✔ Pick up a new hobby.

✔ Discover new music.

✔ Schedule time off.

✔ Schedule alone time.

✔ Schedule fun/play time.

Sometimes taking the path of least resistance is easy, getting into the routine of working, sleeping and watching TV. But ask yourself what else your heart is longing for. How can you sweeten up your life in other areas besides with food?

Part V

The Part of Tens

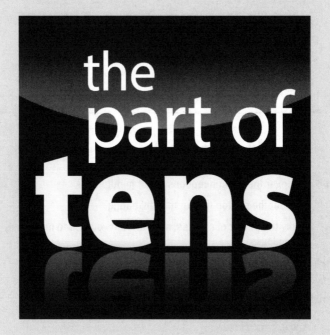

Find an additional Part of Tens chapter on the top ten lessons mindful eating can teach you about life at www.dummies. com/extras/mindfuleating.

In this part . . .

✔ Discover the misconceptions about mindfulness.

✔ Find out the top ten tips for mindful eating.

✔ Apply the power of mindlessness to train yourself to mindlessly eating less.

✔ Explore more ways in which you can continue to practice mindfulness and mindful eating.

Chapter 14

Ten (or so) Misconceptions about Mindfulness

● ●

In This Chapter

▶ Overcoming mental barriers to practicing mindfulness

▶ Recognizing misconceptions about mindfulness

▶ Understanding core concepts of mindfulness

● ●

*M*indfulness is not what you think – literally! Don't let your misconceptions about mindfulness prevent you from diving in. This chapter dispels some of the most common misconceptions about mindfulness. Do you recognize yourself holding on to any of the following beliefs about mindfulness?

I Can't Stop Thinking! Am I Doing It Wrong?

Many people assume that when they sit down to meditate they'll feel this wave of bliss pass over them and all thoughts, cares and desires will fade away with each out-breath. Wouldn't that be nice? But when people actually sit down and tune into what's going on in their minds, they're shocked at how chaotic it can be up there!

If you've ever sat in meditation, even if it was only for as little as 60 seconds, then you probably came to the same conclusion that most people do – stopping thinking is quite challenging! No one can simply flick a switch and make their minds go blank – and that's quite all right. Virtually everyone who starts practicing mindfulness awareness or other forms of meditation immediately notices their busy mind, so if you've noticed this as well, just remember that you're not alone.

The good news is that noticing how busy your mind can be is a great step in the right direction, and it certainly doesn't mean you're not doing it correctly – it actually means you're on the right path. Minds wander; that's just what they do, and the more you practice being aware of your thoughts without attaching to them, the more spaciousness, peace and freedom you'll find in your life.

Eventually, the more you practice, the more you'll have days when you do notice your mind is quieter and more relaxed. This happens because you start to notice the space between your thoughts and explore those gaps. You'll see that this is part of your quiet mind, as opposed to your busy mind. You'll discover the stillness and peace that this spaciousness can offer you.

The Purpose of Mindfulness Is to Go Blank and Not Think

The practice of mindfulness is not about trying to stop or prevent thoughts. It's actually quite the opposite: mindfulness is about loosening the vise-like grip of control and simply allowing your random thoughts to arise and observing them with an unbiased perspective.

The key difference is that with mindfulness, you're cultivating the capacity to observe without getting hooked, lost in or swept away by thoughts. You gradually learn not to resist the thoughts or experiences you don't like and grasp or cling to the ones you do like, but rather to welcome all thoughts and experiences equally (which can be very challenging to do!). When practicing mindfulness, try to think of thoughts as clouds passing in the sky; simply look and watch without judgment as the unbiased observer.

I'm Not Any Good at It!

You'll be happy to hear that most people are able to improve their capacity to pay attention. I hear many people say that they don't know what they're doing, they can't stop thinking or they think it's too simple, so they automatically think they're not very good at it! But practicing mindfulness is not something you're good or bad at. Mindfulness is an inherent ability in all humans that you can practice strengthening.

Remember that if you're like most people, you've also been cultivating your busy mind and distracted mind for most of your life; strengthening the quality of mindfulness takes time and dedication. People practice mindfulness for years and still encounter challenges. But remember, the benefits are well worth it!

It's a Cult/It's a Religion/It's Against Religion/It's Spiritual

Although the formal development of mindfulness meditation practice has its roots in Buddhism and stretches back over 2,500 years, mindfulness has no religious component that you need to adhere to in order to practice it. Focusing your mind and paying attention is a fundamental human gift that transcends all belief systems. Anyone with any belief system can enjoy the many benefits that mindfulness has to offer.

It's So Simple, It Must Be Easy

The instructions for mindfulness meditation are extremely simple, but I hate to break it to you – no one ever said it would be easy! Despite how simple it sounds ('All I have to do is just sit there and pay attention?'), mindfulness can still be quite challenging to practice at times. Don't be fooled by its simplicity! Mindfulness has enough depth to keep you busy practicing for a lifetime!

On the other hand, it doesn't *have* to be challenging, and the mind usually makes it more challenging than it actually is. Mindfulness can be fun, simple and easy if you let go of all attachment, become an unbiased observer and become totally accepting of impermanence and the transient nature of reality! No problem, right?

It's the Answer to All My Problems

Mindfulness may not answer all the secret mysteries of life or solve your most troubling problems, but it can be a helpful and powerful tool to help you reduce stress, start to eat more mindfully, sleep better, improve moods and reverse disease (shall I go on?). Practicing mindfulness helps create an upward spiral that reaches out and influences other areas of your life in a positive way.

Mindfulness can also offer you skills to help you address life's challenges and navigate difficult situations in a positive and constructive way rather than distracting, avoiding or numbing out with food (or watching TV, smoking, shopping . . .).

Mindfulness Is about Running Away from Reality

Mindfulness is not about running away, but rather about facing up to what you may not want to face up to. It's actually a very powerful technique for preventing the habitual knee-jerk reaction of avoiding or distracting yourself from the present moment – something everyone does. That's why it takes a lot of courage to practice mindfulness day in and day out, because you're so accustomed to running away from what you don't want to feel, and mindfulness offers a technique to face these feelings and lean into them, rather than running away from them.

Mindfulness Has No Credibility; It's Just a Passing Fad

All kinds of professionals, from doctors and physical therapists to psychologists and counselors are implementing the use of mindfulness meditation in their practices to help people in all sorts of different ways. Mindfulness has been shown to help people cope with stress and chronic pain, and reduce anxiety and depression.

In the UK, the National Institute for Clinical Excellence (NICE) recommends mindfulness as a treatment for depression, and the American Heart Association recommends using mindfulness as a method to prevent overeating.

When you consider the overwhelming amount of credible research documenting the effectiveness of mindfulness that has already emerged in the past decade and that continues to grow, you can count on seeing the increased use of mindfulness as a recommended antidote to many of today's common ailments.

You Have to Sit Down to Be Mindful

You can practice mindfulness in many ways. Although traditional mindfulness meditations typically involve sitting or walking meditations, you can combine mindfulness practice with anything you do by simply paying more attention, engaging all your senses and focusing on the task at hand. Practicing yoga is also a wonderful way to engage in mindful movement.

I Don't Have Time for Mindfulness

Contrary to what most people believe, when you're engaged in an activity it doesn't actually take much more time to be mindful than it does to be mindless and not pay attention. Formal mindfulness practice (in the form of meditation) does require carving out some time from your busy schedule; can you start to spare ten minutes at some point in your day? Ironically enough, the busiest people with the most hectic, chaotic schedules are the ones who can benefit the most from taking a break from the rush to simply let go, focus and relax their minds.

When you can take the time to practice relaxing your mind, you notice that you can actually concentrate better and become even more productive throughout your day. So instead of thinking, *I don't have time*, think: *I can't afford not to!*

Mindfulness Equals Physical Discomfort

When you think of someone sitting in meditation, do you imagine a slender yogi sitting there twisted up like a pretzel? This myth addresses a common misconception of the formal practice of mindfulness meditation. The purpose of practicing sitting meditation is not to be in agony. Even though traditional styles of mindfulness meditation involve sitting, many people find sitting cross-legged on the floor quite uncomfortable and even downright painful. The purpose of meditation is to become aware of what you're feeling in the present moment. If what you're noticing is a feeling of pain, you don't have to endure it! Mindfulness doesn't mean not moving. If you're feeling discomfort, simply adjust your position in a way that feels better for you. Perhaps you find sitting in a chair or lying down preferable.

Due to the nature of our busy minds and the challenge of trying to sit still, notice if you're using fidgeting, scratching, twitching or swatting at every insect as a means of distraction. Notice what it feels like to experience discomfort or to have an itch without scratching it. The more you can do this and simply notice without reacting, the more you can practice and prevent your knee-jerk reaction to turn to food as a means of distraction when you're not hungry.

You Have to Meditate to Practice Mindfulness

In case you're squirming at the thought of sitting in formal mindfulness meditation, you don't need to sit in meditation to practice mindfulness. Meditation is extremely beneficial and highly recommended, but of course it's not mandatory. Every single moment of every day is a new and wonderful moment to practice mindfulness. Because simply stating, 'I'm going to be mindful of every moment from here on out,' is not realistic, choosing specific activities to practice and foster mindfulness does help, whether it's sitting down on a cushion, chopping vegetables or sitting down to a nice meal. For more information on the formal practice of mindfulness meditation, see *Mindfulness For Dummies* (Wiley, 2010) by Shamash Alidina.

Chapter 15

Top Ten Tips for Mindful Eating

In This Chapter

▶ Discovering simple tips to slow down while eating

▶ Implementing mindful eating tips alone or with others

▶ Reminding yourself to practice mindful eating

*W*ant some easy and fun mindful eating tips to incorporate into your daily routine? In this chapter are ten quick and easy ways to incorporate mindfulness while eating, whether you are alone or with others. These tips are simple yet powerful reminders to slow down and engage with the experience of eating. For best results, implement them on a daily basis!

Sit Down (but Not in the Car)

Although mindfulness is by no means only associated with sitting down, practicing mindful eating is often easier while sitting at a table. When you eat while standing, for the most part, you're usually multitasking, grazing on countertop leftovers or eating on the run – which makes it a lot more challenging to be mindful! Sitting down encourages you to slow down and take the time to tune into the process of eating.

There is a caveat to this guideline – one place you don't want to be sitting while eating is in the car! According to food journalist Michael Pollan, in the US about 20 percent of food is eaten in the car. Eating mindfully is hard when you should be paying attention to your driving! Multitasking while eating increases the likelihood of mindless eating. Sitting down to eat without distractions is a simple way to build a strong foundation for mindful eating.

Pause Before You Eat (Breathe, Smell and Give Thanks!)

Pausing before you eat sounds so simple, yet interrupting the momentum of a rumbling tummy or strong cravings can be extremely difficult. Whether you're feeling that underlying momentous energy driving you to eat or you're simply about to sit down for a snack, remind yourself to pause before you eat, even if it's only for five seconds. Pausing acts as a speed bump to help slow you down and tune you into what you're feeling in your body. Some ways that you can pause are by taking a few deep breaths and really exploring the smell and sight of your food or by giving thanks with a mealtime blessing.

Become a Leftie, or a Rightie

Eating in a way that you're not habitually used to, like eating with your opposite hand, encourages you to pay attention – watch out for that sauce on your white shirt though! When you become accustomed to doing something, it becomes a habit and then oftentimes you no longer pay attention to what you're doing, leading to all kinds of multitasking maneuvers like eating while texting on the phone, watching a movie or reading the paper. Getting out of your normal routine – like eating with the hand that you're not used to – helps kick-start your mindful awareness around food and encourages you to pay attention.

Want to make your dinner parties more fun and incorporate mindful eating at the same time? Watch and giggle as you witness your guests awkwardly eat with chopsticks with their non-dominant hand, which is the left hand for about 90 percent of people. You'll immediately notice everyone's awareness of their eating process perk right up!

This playful mindful eating technique doesn't have to be used only with others – you can also use this method to slow down your own eating when you're alone.

Chew, Chew, Chew Your Food

How often have you heard your mom say: 'Don't forget to chew your food!'? She's got a point on this one. Research shows a correlation between increased chewing and reducing overall food intake. Could it really be that easy? Yes! But it does require being mindful of chewing and remembering to take your time.

Have you ever noticed that food marketers are making food easier and easier to chew? Some people are calling today's packaged and processed foods pre-chewed! Food manufactures want to make it as easy for you as possible to gulp down their food and don't want to put something as tedious as chewing between you and their products. But after implementing the guidelines to healthy eating outlined in Chapter 6, you're now on your way to eating a whole-foods diet that most definitely requires thorough chewing! Chewing is one of the ways that you activate the specific enzymes required to digest your food. By breaking down food to a smooth consistency rather than gulping down large chunks of food, you're lending a helping hand (or set of teeth) to your digestion process.

Count how many times you typically chew your food and then try to add at least ten chews on to it. See if you can notice the way the flavors change in your mouth the longer you chew.

Brake between Bites

Have you ever noticed yourself shoveling more food into your mouth before you even swallowed your last bite? Many people find it hard to slow down, even when they notice how fast they're eating. Practicing braking between bites also helps encourage you to chew your food.

Eating in a rush means you don't have time to enjoy your food, especially when you're focused on your next bite before you've finished the one that's in your mouth! Pausing between bites or even implementing a longer pause midway through the meal allows you to prolong the enjoyment of your food. Reminding yourself to put on the brakes and pause between bites helps you to eat more mindfully. Remind yourself to put down your knife and fork, spoon, or chopsticks and really savor the bite of food you're experiencing.

Taking the time to pause is such a simple technique that's it often forgotten. Slowing down while eating (and slowing down in general!) can help reduce and relieve stress and improve digestion.

When eating with other people, try to eat slower than the slowest eater at the table.

Eat in Silence for at Least Two Minutes

Social events are prime territory for mindless eating. Even the seemingly simple task of engaging in conversation can divert your attention away from the experience of eating and can prompt mindless overeating or undereating.

If you're attending or hosting a social gathering, kindly invite all the guests to eat in silence for the first few minutes of the meal. (You may want to run this by the host before you do!) This method can be a powerful way of minimizing distraction and allowing in more space for mindfulness of the eating process. It allows for a shared time where everyone can participate in mindful eating in a common space.

If you want to practice this one on your own you don't necessarily need everyone else's participation – but you may want to let your eating companions next to you know beforehand, otherwise they may just take you to be a rude guest! Sometimes just tuning out of the conversation for a moment and tuning into your eating experience helps guide you to eating the right amount, especially if you're accustomed to overeating at social events.

Take the First Three Bites with Your Eyes Closed

One way you can practice mindful eating is by taking the time to explore the food in front of you by keeping your eyes closed for the first three mouthfuls. Alternatively you can eat with a blindfold on during your meal.

Your eyes are one of the ways that you engage with and participate in the world around you. But by constantly looking and watching others and the external world you can forget to tune into your inner reality and what you're feeling within yourself and your body. By closing your eyes, you immediately shift your awareness within. When people eat with a blindfold they naturally eat less than they otherwise would, which just goes to show how often you eat with your eyes!

By shutting down or tuning out of one sense, your other senses become sharper as they naturally try to compensate for the loss of the other sense. You may want to try closing your eyes to explore mindfulness of your other senses, such as how your food smells or how it tastes, and also use it as a way to tune into your hunger levels.

Make It Special

Taking the time to make a meal look nice is one of the ways you can nourish yourself through eating. Even though it doesn't have anything to do with the actual calories or nutrients that go into your body, you can still be nourished mentally, emotionally and spiritually by a pleasant experience of food.

Even if you're eating takeout food that you bring home after a long day at work, make an effort to put it on a nice plate, use visually appealing placemats or light a candle and play some enjoyable, relaxing music while you eat. Do you notice a difference in how you experience your meal? Do you pay more attention to the details of your food when you make the meal a more enjoyable experience?

You intuitively make some level of association between how you experience the taste of food and how it's presented. Even if you know it actually makes no difference at all, subconsciously, you think it does!

Stage Habitual Reminders

One of the top reasons most people fail to implement mindful eating into their daily routines is simply because they forget! As you live in a culture where you're constantly using all kinds of automated reminders, why not set a few of them to remind yourself to eat more mindfully?

Find out what reminders work best for you by playing with a few of the following suggestions. You can use written reminders placed on your fridge door, your bathroom mirror or even in your wallet, or digital reminders that you can set at your regular mealtime that chime before you start eating to remind you to slow down, chew your food, brake between bites or practice the body scan before you start to eat (Chapter 8 describes the body scan technique). Be creative and set reminders that actually work for you. The more you practice these simple mindful eating techniques, the more you will automatically (but not mindlessly!) incorporate them into your life on a daily basis.

Only Eat When You Eat

If you could remember and implement only one guideline on your mindful eating journey, I would recommend this one: only eat when you eat. This simple yet far-reaching guideline helps you to sit down, slow down, remove distractions, avoid multitasking and remember to focus your attention and awareness on only doing one thing at a time: exploring the experience of eating while you eat.

Chapter 16

(Almost) Ten Ways to Mindlessly Eat Less

*I*f you could find a way to eat less without noticing, would you implement those changes? Well, there is a way – in fact, many ways, and they're easier to incorporate into your day than you may think.

This book is on mindful eating, so why would I hint that you may benefit from engaging in mindless eating habits? Because you're human! No matter how much you practice mindful eating and how much more aware you become around your eating habits, certain mindless tendencies can always trip up even the most mindful of eaters. This chapter offers tips on how you can take mindful action to automatically prevent the mindless tendencies we all have to overeat and actually gear yourself to eat less, but without even noticing!

Rethink Convenience

You're geared towards convenience and naturally gravitate towards the path of least resistance. This tendency is so powerful that it can mostly go unnoticed. The simple act of having to get up for seconds, or open a cupboard door for a snack, can reduce mindless overeating simply because it requires the slightest bit of extra effort.

This effect has been shown in many different studies, including one conducted by Eastern Illinois University researchers. They gave two groups pistachio nuts; one group had to shell the nuts themselves (a relatively easy thing to do) and the other group received the nuts pre-shelled. Guess who ate more? Although both groups rated their fullness and satisfaction levels the same, the group that didn't have to open the shells ate more – almost 100 calories more in that one sitting. Do that on a daily basis and those extra 100 calories turn into an extra 15 pounds per year! Here are a few ways you can rethink convenience:

✔ **Make low-calorie foods the most convenient option:** By simply replacing a box of crackers on the counter with a bowl of apples, oranges or bananas, you make healthier foods more convenient for you and your whole family. Another way you can make healthy foods the most convenient option is to reorganize your fridge so that fresh foods are the easiest to grab. Place fresh fruits and vegetables at the front of your fridge and everything else at the back. You can wash and cut up vegetables like celery or carrot sticks to make them the easiest choice when you're on the go. This works especially well if you have kids.

✔ **Off the counter, out of reach:** If you don't want to be mindlessly munching all day, don't keep food out on the counter, on your desk at the office or in the car – or wherever you spend the majority of your days. Having food out makes it more convenient than having to go looking for it, and only prompts you to eat more.

✔ **Portion out and put away:** Did you know that you can minimize overeating by simply portioning food out on your plate and then putting away the remaining food? Sounds simple – almost too good to be true – but this strategy is highly effective in preventing mindless eating. After you get into the habit of putting the rest of the food away before you sit down to eat, you're less likely to take it all out again to make yourself another plate of food.

Out of Sight, Out of Mind

This tactic is easy for most people to remember, as I'm sure you've heard it before – out of sight, out of mind. If you're willing to make an effort, this strategy works particularly well by reducing visual triggers to mindless eating. Remember that simply seeing food is enough of a trigger to prompt you to eat without actually being hungry.

Try a few of these suggestions to keep foods out of sight and out of mind.

> ✔ Make a list of the foods that trigger you the most and remove them from your cupboards, fridge, house, office, car and everywhere else that may trigger you.

> ✔ If your favorite TV shows are packed with food commercials, make it a habit to get up and focus on something else whilst the commercial are on.

> ✔ If you're routinely triggered to pull up to a fast-food drive-through or to mindlessly walk into a less-than-healthy restaurant, consider taking an alternative route to avoid the cue.

While avoidance can help, it is not a long-term solution to your eating problems. Addressing your eating habits at their core with mindfulness is crucial to achieve long-lasting change.

In Sight, after the Bite

The one occasion when keeping food in sight helps trigger you to eat less is after you've eaten. How so? If you keep the remnants of a snack or meal in sight, like pistachio shells, chicken wing bones, wrappers, beer bottles or wine glasses, the sight of these items automatically triggers you to consume less. When in sight, these food or beverage leftovers act as powerful visual reminders of how much you've already consumed. Out of sight, out of mind prompts you to forget what you've already consumed, but when the leftovers are in sight, your brain can't deny the evidence lying right in front of it.

Downsize Your Dishware

Did you know that the average household plate continues to get bigger and bigger? A typical household once used an 8- or 9-inch plate, but this average has now stretched to about 12 inches wide! Study after study shows that as soon as you grab a bigger plate to eat off of, you're sure to load more calories onto it – without consciously thinking about it. This optical illusion tricks the brain each and every time, even when you're aware of the bias! When you opt for a larger plate, the same amount of food looks a lot less than when it's on a smaller plate, and your brain registers less food, which typically equals less satisfying. You're geared to always go for more food as opposed to less food as part of your built-in capacity for survival.

Keep your larger plates for low-calorie fruit- and vegetable-based meals like salads and fruit plates, but downsize to smaller dishware for everything else.

Tall and Skinny (versus Short and Wide)

Most people aren't aware of how many calories they consume through beverages in a day.

One way you can mindlessly drink less is if you choose a tall and skinny glass versus a short and wide one. Your mind is geared to notice vertical distance more than horizontal, so a vertical line always looks longer than a horizontal one.

Look at Figure 16-1 and choose the longer line.

This is a trick question because both lines are the same length, yet if you chose the vertical line, don't worry, you're not alone. This tendency is so powerful when it comes to pouring that even the most professional pourers – bartenders – consistently pour more into short, wide glasses than tall skinny ones. Ultimately switching to water or a low-calorie beverage to keep you hydrated is best, but in all other cases, replace your short, wide glasses with tall skinny ones and mindlessly drink in fewer calories.

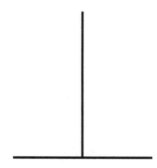

Figure 16-1: Don't always believe your eyes! An optical illusion can make us drink more.

Take Half to Go

Restaurants notoriously serve large portion sizes. Some restaurant meals even pack enough calories to last you a whole day – if not more!

One mindless habit you can implement is to immediately ask for a takeout container (or go green and bring your own), and as soon as your meal comes, package half of it for another meal or give to a friend, family member or even someone hungry on the street.

Saving a Dime Is Bad for Your Waistline: Don't Buy in Bulk

In today's world, you're always trying to figure out ways to economize and save a few bucks, especially when it comes to rising food prices. Although buying in bulk may save you a few extra dollars here and there, you're way more likely to eat more when you have more bulk food in the house.

> ✔ Store bulk and excess packages somewhere other than the kitchen, like the garage or basement, in a dry, clean storage space. Keep the bulk food out of sight and out of mind to help reduce the constant visual cues that can prompt you to mindlessly eat more.

✔ If you do continue to buy in bulk, portion out smaller serving sizes into a resealable bag or plastic container to keep on hand in the kitchen and leave the rest in another storage space.

✔ Don't eat from the package – especially if it's of the super-size variety. Portion food onto a plate or bowl so that you can see how much you're eating in one sitting and then put the rest of the package away.

The best foods to buy in bulk are healthy foods like fruits and vegetables.

Downsize the Display (Minimize Variety)

Did you know that the more variety you sit down to at any given meal, the more likely you are to overeat? That's why buffets set the stage for one of the most common mindless eating (and often overeating) scenarios.

Whether you're having guests over for dinner or are making food for the family, find a healthy balance between too much and too little variety. When eating out at a buffet or a friend's house, try to put no more than three foods on your plate at a time.

Discover Your Mindless Margin

The *mindless margin* is a term coined by Dr. Brian Wansink, a consumer psychologist and professor at Cornell University, and refers to how you can mindlessly consume less food without being aware of it. Eating only a couple of hundred fewer calories than usual on a daily basis leaves you still feeling satisfied, and, most importantly, avoids feelings of deprivation, but making small changes that seem negligible add up over time, and you're able to lose weight without even noticing.

A mindless margin habit can be something like downsizing your dishware or putting the food away after you portion out your meal. All the suggestions offered in this chapter fall within this category. When you get into an eating habit that automatically prevents you from overeating, you're using the power of mindlessness to work in your favor.

Chapter 17

Ten Paths to Expand Your Mindful Eating Experience

*W*ant to keep exploring new paths for mindful eating or mindfulness in general? Explore these top ten paths to expand your experience and continue to grow, develop and flourish on your mindfulness path.

Become a Member of the Center for Mindful Eating

The Center for Mindful Eating, also known as TCME, is led by a diverse board of trained professionals and is geared towards helping other professionals, institutions and the general public implement the principles and practices of mindful eating.

This website offers abundant information through articles, a free newsletter and teleconferences, and also offers additional resources to paid members, with a discount for current students. These members-only resources are especially aimed at educating health-oriented professionals on the principles of mindfulness to better serve their clients.

But don't worry! You don't have to become a member to benefit from their online resources. Check out their website at www.thecenterformindfuleating.org.

Start a Mindful Eating Group

Want some company as you embark on your mindful eating journey? Invite your friends and family and start a weekly or monthly mindful eating group.

You have a lifetime of both mindful and mindless eating experiences to share with others. And just as you have something to share on this topic, usually others do as well – which makes for a perfect group dynamic where everyone can learn from each other! In this way, everyone becomes both teacher and student.

Don't worry if you don't feel qualified to lead a group like this. Take a leap of faith! You'll be amazed at how much you can discover about your own relationship with food through discussing it in a group setting.

If you want to extend the group beyond your friends and family by inviting the public, explore some of the great online websites that help bring people together with similar interests – although you may not want to host the group at your own home. Check out MeetUp (www.meetup.com) and search in your area to see if there's already a mindful eating group that you can join, or if you want to start one, go right ahead and take the lead!

Get One-on-One Coaching

If you have some more serious eating challenges that you'd like to discuss with a professional, consider getting one-on-one coaching or counseling. With the increased popularity of mindful eating, more healthcare professionals are integrating it into their practices and offering mindful eating coaching as part of their services.

If you are struggling with an eating disorder, please consult a doctor.

The Center for Mindful Eating has a 'Find a Professional' tab on its website and offers a list of healthcare professionals.

Attend a Mindful Eating Retreat

Finding it a little difficult to incorporate mindful eating into your everyday routine at home? Maybe you have a family to feed or have to hurry around in the morning helping your kids get ready for school? If this sounds like you, you're probably in need of a vacation! Why not take a vacation to a beautiful beach or tropical paradise *and* explore mindful eating at the same time?

We offer mindful eating retreats here in Hawaii (see www. happyandraw.com), and many other options are available.

Mindfulness-Based Eating Awareness Training (MB-EAT), developed by clinical psychologist Professor Jean Kristeller, is a great choice. You can find listings of upcoming MB-EAT retreats at the Center for Mindful Eating website: www. thecenterformindfuleating.org.

The Zen Community of Oregon occasionally hosts mindful eating retreats with Jan Chozen Bays, author of *Mindful Eating: A Guide to Rediscovering a Healthy and Joyful Relationship with Food* (Shambhala) and co-founder of the Great Vow Zen Monastery. See the website www.zendust.org for more details on upcoming events.

Attend a Mindfulness Retreat

Although mindfulness retreats aren't focused solely on mindful eating, they are focused on mindful living, which of course, incorporates awareness around eating. Several well-known places offer mindfulness retreats, including:

> ✔ **Vipassana Ten-day Retreats:** These retreats can be a profound, life-changing experience and are now held all over the world. You arrive at a specific location and practice various forms of meditation, all in silence – and I mean *all* in silence; participants don't speak for the whole ten days. This retreat may sound daunting, and, yes, it is

challenging, but the retreat can offer you an extremely valuable opportunity to help benefit many areas of your life, including helping mend an unhealthy relationship to food. See the website www.dhamma.org/en/index for more information about ten-day retreats offered in your area.

✔ **Plum Village**: Located in France and founded by spiritual teacher and peace activist Thich Nhat Hanh, Plum Village offers mindfulness retreats throughout the year. See the website at www.plumvillage.org for more information.

✔ **Gampo Abbey**: Gampo Abbey is a Buddhist monastery in Nova Scotia, Canada that offers short in-house retreats. See www.gampoabbey.org for more information.

Take a Course on Mindfulness

Mindfulness is no passing fad, and the courses offered in mindfulness training are getting more and more popular.

✔ One of the people who helped popularize mindfulness is Dr. Jon Kabat-Zinn, founder of Mindfulness-Based Stress Reduction (MBSR), which is taught as an eight-week training course. Dr. Kabat-Zinn also offers a seven-day training course for professionals called Mindfulness-Based Stress Reduction in Mind-Body Medicine. See the website www.umassmed.edu/cfm/7day/index.aspx for more information.

✔ Many people are now trained to teach the MBSR course, and with the power of the web you can now participate in an MBSR course from the comfort of your very own home through the company eMindful. A one-session mindful eating course is also available from eMindful. Check out the website www.emindful.com for the full range of courses offered.

✔ Sounds True (www.soundstrue.com) offers a wide range of audio courses, including one of my favorites, *How to Meditate with Pema Chödrön*.

The following websites also offer a range of courses and retreats on mindfulness:

✔ Naropa University: www.naropa.edu

✔ Insight Meditation Society: www.dharma.org

✔ Upaya Zen Center: www.upaya.org

✔ Shambhala: www.shambhala.org/

Keep a Mindful Eating Journal

Writing provides another outlet to help mentally register and lock in what you're discovering about mindful eating. It helps create new habits as you visually see the insights and experiences you've had staring back at you on the page. A journal is another way that you can remind yourself why mindless eating hasn't been working for you and why mindful eating is a better direction to head in. Your journal will offer invaluable insights, be a trusted companion and help to encourage you on your path.

Taking the time to reflect and write about mindful eating also offers you another method to emotionally process challenges around your relationship with your food, your eating, your body and even your life. And on top of that, keeping a mindful eating journal can also be a mindfulness practice in its own right!

Don't forget to check out Chapter 4 for more on keeping a mindful eating journal.

Grow Your Mindfulness Library

One way to help remind yourself to keep practicing mindful eating is to keep reading about it! Many books out there focus specifically on mindful eating, and others offer a wider view of mindfulness practice in everyday living.

Head over to www.amazon.com and search for 'mindfulness' or 'mindful eating' and see what comes up. Read book descriptions, author bios and reviews and choose the books that you resonate with the most.

Stay Mindfully Connected with Websites and Social Media

With the growing popularity of social media, why not use social media to help you focus on your goals, like starting to eat more mindfully? Hundreds of Facebook pages are geared towards mindfulness. By going in and clicking 'like' on these pages, you're basically asking to see their daily posts in your own news feed, so you can effortlessly be exposed to a daily dose of affirmations, quotes, resources, good advice and all things mindfulness.

Most of the time, when you find a website you like you can see a social media icon on the webpage. By clicking that icon, you link right to its social media page, whether it's on Facebook, Twitter, Pinterest, YouTube, Google+ or one of the many other social media sites.

Use Technology to Support Mindfulness

If you own a cell phone you can set automatic reminders to prompt (and train) yourself to become more mindful in the moment. Two main ways you can do this are:

- ✔ Set a specific soft and gentle sound to ding or ring at three different times throughout the day, especially around meal times. Make this your mindfulness sound so that you can start to train yourself to tune into the present moment every time you hear the ding. This sound helps whether you're eating or not. When you hear that sound, take a moment to stop what you're doing, tune into your body and take a few deep, mindful breaths.

- ✔ You can also set more specific reminders around mindful eating that send you actual messages like 'slow down', 'pause' and 'chew your food'. You can set these reminders to repeat every day and also change them based on what you want to focus on for the week.

Index

About the Author

Laura Dawn is a Registered Holistic Nutritionist (RHN). A whole-foods chef, mindful eating mentor and avid organic gardener, Laura is also a dynamic workshop presenter and speaker. By inspiring people to drop their struggle with food and weight, Laura helps people reconnect to the sacredness of food and their inner body wisdom and reach optimal health by transitioning to a real foods lifestyle. Her passion is to inspire others to develop a healthy relationship to food, to their bodies and to Mother Earth.

Founder of the website Happy & Raw (www.happyandraw. com), Laura facilitates health retreats and internship programs on the Big Island of Hawaii, where she currently resides.

Dedication

This book is dedicated to you, the reader, and the many millions of people who struggle with food and eating whom I aspire to help with the power of mindful eating.

May mindful eating support you on your journey to health and wellness and help you cultivate a truly profound relationship with food, your body and this earth.

Author's Acknowledgments

Heartfelt gratitude to all those at John Wiley & Sons, Inc., for helping bring this book to fruition. I would like to personally thank Michelle Hacker for stepping in to support this project with the most perfect timing; Andrew Kennerley, for supporting me through this project; Sarah Blankfield, who initially invited me to write this book; and Rachael Chilvers, who contributed a helping hand along the way.

I would like to express sincere gratitude to Jon Kabat-Zinn and Pema Chödrön, neither of whom I've met (yet), but I carry them and their profound teachings on mindfulness close to my heart. Both of their lives' work has strongly influenced my own personal and professional life. On that note, I would also like to extend a special acknowledgment to the Center for Mindful Eating (www.thecenterformindfuleating.org) and all the wonderful mindful eating resources that they offer the public.

And, finally, saying a simple 'thank you' to both my husband and mother for all their support could never quite cover the level of gratitude I feel for having them in my life. Noah, it's amazing how hard you work to make space and afford me the opportunity to write. I am eternally grateful for you. And Lucy, I wouldn't be where I am if it weren't for you.

Publisher's Acknowledgments

Acquisitions Editor: Andrew Kennerley

Project Manager: Michelle Hacker

Project Editors: Rachael Chilvers, Simon Bell

Development Editor: Martin Key

Copy Editor: Kelly Cattermole

Technical Editor: Sophie Roberts, RD

Project Coordinator: Sheree Montgomery

Cover Image: ©iStock.com/gerenme

Take Dummies with you everywhere you go!

Whether you're excited about e-books, want more from the web, must have your mobile apps, or swept up in social media, Dummies makes everything easier.

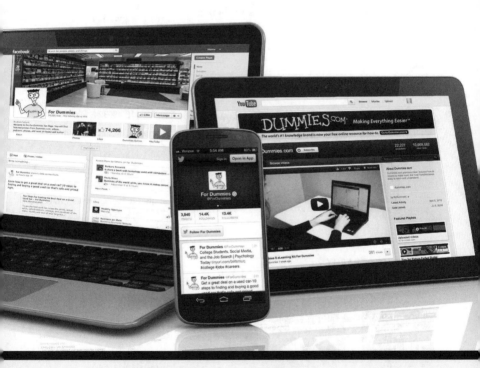

FOR DUMMIES®

A Wiley Brand

BUSINESS

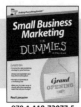

Small Business Marketing For Dummies
978-1-118-73077-5

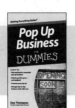

Pop Up Business For Dummies
978-1-118-44349-1

Starting & Running a Business All-in-One For Dummies
978-1-119-97527-4

MUSIC

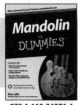

Mandolin For Dummies
978-1-119-94276-4

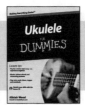

Ukulele For Dummies
978-0-470-97799-6

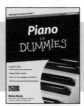

Piano For Dummies
978-0-470-49644-2

DIGITAL PHOTOGRAPHY

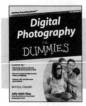

Digital Photography For Dummies
978-1-118-09203-3

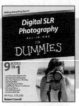

Digital SLR Photography All-in-One For Dummies
978-0-470-76878-5

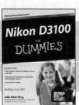

Nikon D3100 For Dummies
978-1-118-00472-2

Algebra I For Dummies
978-0-470-55964-2

Anatomy & Physiology For Dummies, 2nd Edition
978-0-470-92326-9

Asperger's Syndrome For Dummies
978-0-470-66087-4

Basic Maths For Dummies
978-1-119-97452-9

Body Language For Dummies, 2nd Edition
978-1-119-95351-7

Bookkeeping For Dummies, 3rd Edition
978-1-118-34689-1

British Sign Language For Dummies
978-0-470-69477-0

Cricket for Dummies, 2nd Edition
978-1-118-48032-8

Currency Trading For Dummies, 2nd Edition
978-1-118-01851-4

Cycling For Dummies
978-1-118-36435-2

Diabetes For Dummies, 3rd Edition
978-0-470-97711-8

eBay For Dummies, 3rd Edition
978-1-119-94122-4

Electronics For Dummies All-in-One For Dummies
978-1-118-58973-1

English Grammar For Dummies
978-0-470-05752-0

French For Dummies, 2nd Edition
978-1-118-00464-7

Guitar For Dummies, 3rd Edition
978-1-118-11554-1

IBS For Dummies
978-0-470-51737-6

Keeping Chickens For Dummies
978-1-119-99417-6

Knitting For Dummies, 3rd Edition
978-1-118-66151-2